100 Questions & Answers
About Endometriosis

David B. Redwine, MD, FACOG

Medical Director
Endometriosis Institute of Oregon
St. Charles Medical Center
Bend, Oregon

JONES AND BARTLETT PUBLISHERS
Sudbury, Massachusetts
BOSTON   TORONTO   LONDON   SINGAPORE

World Headquarters

Jones and Bartlett Publishers
40 Tall Pine Drive
Sudbury, MA 01776
978-443-5000
info@jbpub.com
www.jbpub.com

Jones and Bartlett Publishers
Canada
6339 Ormindale Way
Mississauga, Ontario L5V 1J2
Canada

Jones and Bartlett Publishers
International
Barb House, Barb Mews
London W6 7PA
United Kingdom

Jones and Bartlett's books and products are available through most bookstores and online booksellers. To contact Jones and Bartlett Publishers directly, call 800-832-0034, fax 978-443-8000, or visit our website, www.jbpub.com.

Substantial discounts on bulk quantities of Jones and Bartlett's publications are available to corporations, professional associations, and other qualified organizations. For details and specific discount information, contact the special sales department at Jones and Bartlett via the above contact information or send an email to specialsales@jbpub.com.

The authors, editor, and publisher have made every effort to provide accurate information. However, they are not responsible for errors, omissions, or for any outcomes related to the use of the contents of this book and take no responsibility for the use of the products and procedures described. Treatments and side effects described in this book may not be applicable to all people; likewise, some people may require a dose or experience a side effect that is not described herein. Drugs and medical devices are discussed that may have limited availability controlled by the Food and Drug Administration (FDA) for use only in a research study or clinical trial. Research, clinical practice, and government regulations often change the accepted standard in this field. When consideration is being given to use of any drug in the clinical setting, the healthcare provider or reader is responsible for determining FDA status of the drug, reading the package insert, and reviewing prescribing information for the most up-to-date recommendations on dose, precautions, and contraindications, and determining the appropriate usage for the product. This is especially important in the case of drugs that are new or seldom used.

Production Credits

Executive Publisher: Christopher Davis
Editorial Assistant: Jessica Acox
Production Editor: Rachel Rossi
Production Intern: Ashlee Hazeltine
Associate Marketing Manager: Ilana Goddess
V.P., Manufacturing and Inventory Control:
   Therese Connell
Composition: Spoke & Wheel/Jason Miranda

Cover Design: Kristin E. Ohlin
Cover Image: Top Left: ©Trilobite/Dreamstime.com;
   Top Right: © Petarneychev/Dreamstime.com;
   Bottom Left: © Iofoto/Dreamstime.com; Bottom
   Right: © Sorinus/Dreamstime.com
Printing and Binding: Malloy, Inc.
Cover Printing: Malloy, Inc.

Library of Congress Cataloging-in-Publication Data
Redwine, David B.
   100 questions & answers about endometriosis / David B. Redwine.
      p. cm.
   ISBN-13: 978-0-7637-5923-0 (alk. paper)
   ISBN-10: 0-7637-5923-6 (alk. paper)
   1. Endometriosis—Popular works. 2. Endometriosis—Miscellanea. I. Title. II. Title: 100 questions and answers about endometriosis. III. Title: One hundred questions and answers about endometriosis.
   RG483.E53R43 2009
   618.1—dc22   3061
                                            2008036078
6048

Printed in the United States of America
12 11 10 09 08   10 9 8 7 6 5 4 3 2 1

This book is dedicated to patients with endometriosis, all of whom have had an incredible impact on my life.

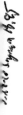

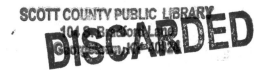

CONTENTS

Endometriosis is one of the most commonly seen gynecological diseases and continues to be poorly misunderstood by both physicians and patients alike. It is a potent cause of pelvic pain and can be a cause of infertility. Endometriosis is responsible for hundreds of millions of dollars in expenditures around the world each year, as a result of both direct medical costs and indirect costs related to its interference with life and work.

My interest in the disease is both personal and professional—my first wife had endometriosis. Through her I experienced all of the frustrations that women with the disease and their partners can go through. I was taught in medical school about the confusion surrounding the disease, and experiencing this confusion personally drove home the point that there must be a better way of understanding endometriosis. I just happened to be in a position to observe the disease firsthand in my patients and to see if I could find a better way.

I mentally threw away all the textbook theories on the disease and developed new ways of looking at it, both visually and by using computer database management techniques. I let the disease speak for itself by revealing its true character through these studies. The picture of endometriosis that emerged was completely different from what I'd been taught and what everyone believed. It's been my mission in life ever since to tell the revealed truth about endometriosis, not just repeat the mistakes others had been saying for the last 80 years. Endometriosis becomes readily understandable with this new insight and no longer is a "chronic, enigmatic, incurable" disease. It is potentially curable and preventable with surgery, but the surgery must be complete and performed by a qualified gynecological surgeon with experience in dealing with endometriosis.

This little book is the result of one-third of a century of professional effort directed at understanding and treating endometriosis surgically in more than 3,000 patients. It rejects much of what is considered accepted conventional wisdom about the disease, because that conventional wisdom is promoted by those lacking deep experience with the disease. Conventional wisdom has failed—quite miserably—to produce useful progress in true understanding of the disease, instead comfortably repeating what has been said for generations before. The roots of this failure are easily identifiable and can be named: reliance on a theory of origin that obviously is wrong and over-dependence on drugs marketed by companies interested in making money. Better insight into the disease is available to guide its treatment, and this book will introduce you to the very basics of that approach.

Women with endometriosis go through a lot in their lives. My hope is that this book will mean that some may not have to go through any more of the trials and tribulations that this disease can bring.

David Redwine, M.D.
Bend, Oregon

Endometriosis Past

I've known about endometriosis longer than I care to remember. And I've known Dr. Redwine almost as long. As an RN working at the same hospital where Dr. Redwine works, I attended a talk he gave to the medical staff in the 1980s. I had undergone removal of my pelvic organs as treatment for endometriosis when I was 29. Although my symptoms were better, they weren't entirely gone, and in the back of my mind I wondered if I still had some endometriosis inside me. I sat in the back of the room not expecting much. What I heard blew me away! Dr. Redwine outlined an entirely new way of looking at the disease based on better identification at surgery. It turned out that most endometriosis didn't look like what the textbooks said, so almost everything we thought we knew about the disease had to be wrong. Not only that, he presented a new way of treating it by laparoscopic excision and had a believable theory of origin to boot!

I almost couldn't believe that this information came from a general gynecologist working at a general hospital 110 miles away from the nearest interstate highway in Bend, Oregon. His presentation answered all the questions I had about the disease and explained the confusion that existed then and exists now. I was so fired up I had to do something, so I helped found the St. Charles Endometriosis Treatment Program, the world's first program dedicated to treating endometriosis by aggressive surgical excision. I marveled at the success stories I heard from the patients who came to Bend for surgery, most of whom had had several previous surgeries and several rounds of medical treatment. It seemed miraculous to them, but to me it was common-sense surgery based on common-sense observations. I even heard success stories from patients who had had their pelvic organs removed in previous surgeries but their endometriosis had been left in. They, too, seemed to respond to the common-sense treatment of surgical removal of disease from their bodies. What a concept! Removing disease from the body! When it was finally done, women improved.

I couldn't stand it any longer. I wanted to know if it was true, so I signed up for surgery myself, and you know what? It worked! I felt so lucky. I had helped create a program that not only helped women suffering from a very common disease, but also eventually helped me get rid of my own pain. I'd always been a believer in this program, and I'm an even stronger believer now.

As I read the book that you hold in your hands now, I remembered with pride the story behind the scenes that I was a part of. The truths in this book are the result of the entire career of a surgeon who simply wanted to understand and treat endometriosis better and had the bravery and intelligence to question the status quo and provide better answers—100 of them, actually.

—Nancy F. Petersen, RN

PART ONE

The Basics

What is the endometrium?

What is endometriosis?

Can endometriosis occur in males?

More . . .

1. What is the uterus and what does it do?

The **uterus** (**Figure 1**) is the reproductive organ that carries each of us inside our mothers before we are born. It is roughly the size of a pear in the nonpregnant state and consists of two anatomical parts: the lower opening (**cervix**) and the main body (fundus). The uterus is located down low in the central pelvis, just behind the pubic bone and the bladder. It is mainly composed of muscle and has a smooth, shiny external coating called the serosa.

The uterus has an inner cavity lined by glandular tissue called the **endometrium** (**endo-** means "inside"). Each month, part of this inner **uterine lining** sloughs and sheds, producing the menstrual flow (**menstruation**), which flows through the cervix and into the vagina. When the menstrual flow is brisk, the bloody discharge from the vagina can be bright red and fairly liquid. When the menstrual flow is slower, the bloody discharge can be darker red or black and thicker.

Uterus

The muscular organ that contains and supports the fetus before birth. The uterus has two parts: the upper body (fundus) and the opening (cervix).

Cervix

The opening of the uterus through which menstrual blood passes. The cervix opens during labor and delivery to allow passage of the fetus out of the uterus during birth.

Endometrium

The tissue that lines the uterine cavity.

Endo-

A medical prefix meaning "inside" or "within."

Uterine lining

The interior lining of the uterus; the endometrium. The muscular wall of the uterus is the myometrium.

Menstruation

The monthly discharge from the uterus; consists of blood and endometrium sloughed from the uterine lining.

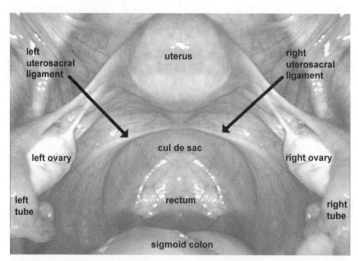

Figure 1 Anatomy of the normal human female pelvis

2. What are the ovaries and what do they do?

There are two **ovaries**, one on each side of the uterus. These whitish structures range in size and shape from about the size of a woman's thumb to a man's thumb. A small ligament connects each ovary to the upper side of the uterus, and each ovary is also connected to the fallopian tube.

The ovary has two main jobs: to produce eggs and to produce the **ovarian hormones—estrogen, progesterone**, and **testosterone**. The ovaries are the storehouses for eggs. The medical term for an egg is **ovum**. At birth, the ovaries carry all the eggs that a woman will ever have, approximately 200,000 in each ovary. New eggs are not produced after birth. Each egg is surrounded by a tiny fluid-filled follicle. After birth, some of the eggs degenerate, so a woman will not necessarily have 400,000 normal eggs for ovulation in her lifetime. Nevertheless, there should be plenty available for ovulation and reproduction.

After puberty, **hormones** from the pituitary gland begin to stimulate the ovary to produce eggs; these eggs have been sitting dormant since birth. Each month, one or more follicles will be "chosen" by hormonal signals to ovulate that month. At that time, the follicle accumulates more fluid within it and expands in size as the egg within that follicle begins to mature and become ready for fertilization. Approximately two weeks after each menstrual flow, a surge of pituitary hormone causes the mature follicle to rupture, releasing the egg in the process called **ovulation**.

Ovary

The repository for ova (eggs) inside the female.

Ovarian hormones

The hormones produced by the ovaries: estrogen, progesterone, and testosterone.

Estrogen

The main hormone produced by the ovaries.

At birth, each ovary contains about 200,000 eggs. Not all of these eggs will be released over the course of a woman's lifetime.

Progesterone

A hormone produced by the ovary, but only if ovulation has occurred. Its action is to prepare the endometrium for implantation of the embryo.

THE BASICS

Testosterone

A male hormone produced by the ovaries around the time of ovulation. It apparently increases the likelihood of mating and fertilization of eggs.

Ovum

The medical term for an egg; plural = ova.

Hormone

A molecule that is produced by one tissue and carried in the bloodstream to another tissue to cause a biological effect.

Ovulation

The release of an ovum by an ovary. Sometimes more than one egg is released at ovulation.

Fallopian tubes

Hollow tubes that pick up eggs that have been released at ovulation and transport those eggs toward the uterus. Fertilization by a sperm occurs within the fallopian tube.

Fimbria

A fringelike part or structure (of the fallopian tube). Plural: fimbriae.

3. What are the fallopian tubes, and what do they do?

There are two **fallopian tubes**, one on each side of the uterus. These very flexible, hollow tubes are approximately 4 inches long and the diameter of a straw; they are attached near the top of the uterus. The hollow cavity of the fallopian tube passes through the side of the uterus and connects with the inner cavity of the uterus. The other end of the fallopian tube is open to the pelvic cavity and has delicate, finger-like tissue at the end, called **fimbriae**.

The fallopian tubes have several jobs. The fimbriae pick up eggs after ovulation. The thin muscular layer in the wall of the tube then begins to "swallow" the egg toward the uterus, in a manner similar to how the esophagus swallows food from the mouth into the stomach. Either tube may pick up eggs from either ovary, not necessarily just an egg from the ovary immediately adjacent to it.

The testosterone surge from the ovaries, which occurs chiefly around the time of ovulation, can cause a female's sex drive to increase, possibly encouraging an episode of sexual intercourse and the deposit of sperm in the vagina next to the cervix. The sperm swim up through the cervix, up the walls of the inner cavity of the uterus, and out the fallopian tubes. If an egg has been swallowed into the far end of one or both fallopian tubes, it may be fertilized by a single sperm.

Fertilization occurs when the DNA from the sperm is combined with the DNA from the egg. It most commonly takes place within an inch of the fimbriated end of the fallopian tube. Over the course of a few days, the fertilized egg continues to divide as it is "swallowed" toward the uterus by the peristaltic action of the fallopian tube. By the time the fertilized egg enters the uterine cavity, it is ready to attach and become implanted in the inner lining of the uterus.

4. What is the endometrium?

The endometrium is the lining of the cavity inside the uterus. It consists of two layers. The functional layer is the part that sloughs and sheds with the menstrual flow, accompanied by bleeding from small arterioles within the lining that break open along with the sloughing outer layer of endometrium. The second layer of the endometrium is a basal layer analogous to the roots of grass, which allows the outer layer to regenerate each month, just like blades of grass regenerate from the roots after each mowing. This basal layer lays against the muscle of the wall of the uterus.

When viewed under the microscope, the endometrial tissue of the endometrium shows a characteristic pattern of glands and stroma. The glands are tiny cystic spaces that are connected by ducts to the inner cavity of the uterus. They secrete a mucus-like material. The glands are surrounded by stroma, which is tissue providing mechanical support and hormonal influence on the glands. The glands and stroma are embedded in connective tissue that holds everything together.

The main job of the endometrium is to accept the implantation of the fertilized egg that drops into the uterine cavity several days after ovulation and to nurture the dividing cells in the early stages of pregnancy. The disease process called endometriosis derives its name from the endometrium.

5. What is endometriosis?

Endometriosis is tissue that somewhat resembles the inner lining of the uterus, but that is located outside of the uterus where it doesn't belong. There are two parts to the word "endometriosis": "endometri" obviously refers to the endometrium lining the inside cavity of the uterus, and "osis" is a generic term for a disease or derangement of a certain type of tissue. Thus the term "endometriosis" refers to a disease or derangement of the endometrium, although this is not quite correct as I'll explain below. Endometriosis consists of glands and stroma. (**Figure 2**)

*Microscopi-
cally, endo-
metriosis is
composed of
two types of
cells: glands
and stroma.
The occur-
rence of both
types of cells
is the "gold
standard" for
diagnosis.*

6. Is endometriosis identical to the endometrium lining the inside of the uterus?

Not at all. It was once thought that endometriosis is exactly identical to the endometrium, but now we know that there are hundreds of basic and profound differences between endometriosis and the endometrium.

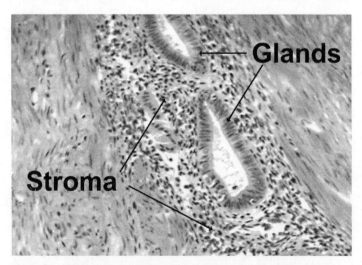

Figure 2 Microscopic appearance of endometriosis showing glands
surrounded by stroma

These differences include genetic differences between the two types of tissue as well as differences in enzymatic activity, **hormone receptors**, hormone responsiveness, microscopic appearance, and visual appearance.

7. How long have doctors known about endometriosis?

Several hundred years ago, some women were known to have a painful condition resulting in "ulcerations" in the pelvis, which were eventually found at autopsy. Because microscopic examination of this tissue was not done at the time, it may or may not have been endometriosis.

The modern history of endometriosis began in the late 1800s. At the turn of the nineteenth century, and for the first two decades of the twentieth century, the disease was known as **adenomyoma**. This name came about because, when examined under the microscope, the abnormal tissue resembled the then-new and interesting disease called adenomyosis of the uterus: The glands and stroma resembling those of the uterine lining were surrounded by newly formed muscle tissue, forming an adeno (*glandular*) myoma (*muscle tumor*). Adenomyomas were reported in the inguinal canal, rectovaginal septum, rectum, and bladder. Today, such adenomyomas would be called deep or invasive endometriosis. Endometriosis was "named" in the 1920s by Dr. John Sampson.

8. How common is endometriosis?

Endometriosis is the leading cause of pelvic pain in women of reproductive age (15 to 40 years of age). We don't know the true percentage of women who have this disease, because it would be necessary to perform surgery

Hormone receptors

Sites on the surface of cells to which hormone molecules attach. The receptor sites are specific to a certain type of hormone. For example, estrogen receptors accept the attachment of estrogen; progesterone receptors accept the attachment of progesterone.

Adenomyoma

The earliest name for what we would now call deep or invasive endometriosis.

to make a definitive diagnosis, whether the women were symptomatic or not. The best guess is that between 1% and 10% of all women have endometriosis. When groups of women with specific symptoms are examined, the prevalence of endometriosis is much higher. For example, in women with **infertility**, approximately 50% are found to have endometriosis; in those with typical pelvic pain and tenderness on pelvic examination, approximately 95% have the disease.

Infertility
The state of being not fertile and unable to become pregnant.

9. What age range does endometriosis affect?

The youngest patient with endometriosis was 10, the oldest was 78.

Tissue resembling endometriosis has been found in the lower pelvis of an infant female dying of sudden infant death syndrome. The youngest living female with endometriosis reported in the literature was just past her tenth birthday when she was diagnosed surgically after only a few menstrual flows. The oldest patient reported with the disease was 78. It is very common for women with endometriosis to have a surgical diagnosis between the ages of 18 and 30 after having suffered symptoms for 8 years or more.

10. What is reflux menstruation?

Sampson thought that endometriosis occurred when refluxed endo-metrial cells or tissue frag-ments invaded the pelvic surfaces.

Normally, the monthly menstrual flow containing both sloughed tissue fragments from the endometrium and blood passes through the cervix and into the vagina. In some women, some of the menstrual discharge backs up in the uterus and begins to reflux or flow out through the fallopian tubes. Most of the menstrual blood still winds up in the vagina, though. When the refluxing blood and tissue reach the open ends of the fallopian tubes, they drip out into the pelvic cavity. This phenomenon is called **reflux menstruation**. Bloody fluid in the pelvic cavity during menstruation may occur in as high as 85% of certain populations of women, such as those undergoing peritoneal dialysis, although the occurrence of bloody fluid doesn't prove that reflux menstruation has occurred. Occasionally during surgical examination of the pelvis during menstruation, blood can be seen coming out the end of the fallopian tubes, although this is an uncommon finding. Fragile capillary beds, which respond to the ovarian hormones by bleeding, can also result in bloody fluid within the pelvis and this type of internal bleeding is not directly related to endometriosis.

Reflux menstruation

Menstrual blood and endometrial tissue flowing in reverse from the uterus out through the fallopian tubes.

THE BASICS

11. Who was Dr. John Sampson?

John Albert Sampson was an American gynecologist who operated a private practice in Albany, New York, in the first half of the twentieth century. His name is synonymous with an old theory of origin of endometriosis.

12. What is the theory of reflux menstruation as the origin of endometriosis?

Sampson suggested that endometriosis occurs as a result of reflux menstruation. According to this theory, endometrial cells and tissue fragments sloughed from the uterine lining during menstruation might sometimes flow against the normal peristaltic action of the fallopian tube. In support of this idea, fragments of sloughed endometrial tissue have occasionally been found within the fallopian tube.

*There is no direct proof of Sampson's theory of origin of endometriosis by photomicrographs, so cartoons are used to illustrate the "missing links. (see **Figure 3**, Page 10)"*

When the cells or tissue fragments that have sloughed from the endometrial lining of the uterus reach the end of the fallopian tubes, they enter the pelvic cavity. In fact, endometrial cells or fragments of sloughed endometrial tissue have been identified in the fluid found in the pelvis in some women.

The theory of reflux menstruation as the origin of endometriosis holds that refluxed cells and tissue fragments that have entered the pelvic cavity then undergo two key steps. First, they attach to pelvic surfaces. Second, they proliferate and invade the surface tissue to become the disease endometriosis. Microscopic evidence for these two key steps has not been found in women with the disease, and all textbook or medical journal article depictions of these two steps are in cartoon format (**Figure 3**).

Autotransplant

Tissue from one area of the body is transplanted surgically or by trauma to another part of the same body. In the new location, the tissue remains identical to tissue formerly in the normal location.

Physicians were once taught that endometriosis was an **autotransplant** (normal tissue transferred from one area of the body to another) identical to the endometrium. As a result, once established, endometriosis should slough and shed and bleed internally just like the endometrium lining the inner uterine cavity, resulting in pain or infertility. In reality, endometriosis does not slough and shed like the menstruating uterine lining and many lesions of endometriosis are not associated with bleeding. The hundreds of differences between endometriosis and the endometrium guarantee that it is not an autotransplant.

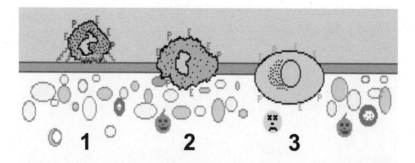

Figure 3 Typical cartoon depiction of the first two missing steps of Sampson's theory. There is plenty of photomicrographic proof of step 3, which is established endometriosis.

It was once thought that women with a weak immune system developed endometriosis because their cellular defense was too weak to fight off refluxed menstrual tissue. Women with endometriosis were imagined to have an unusually high occurrence of infections and autoimmune diseases. However, studies by the Endometriosis Association of women with endometriosis have shown that less than 1% of women with the disease have any other disease that might be considered an autoimmune disease, so there is no proof of an important relationship between the origin of endometriosis and the immune system. In the past, it was also believed that reflux menstruation would occur each month, meaning that increasingly more endometriosis would appear in the pelvis over time, like dandelions spreading in a lawn. Thus the disease was considered incurable, with older women expected to have more pelvic areas of involvement than younger women, although they do not.

Because the theory of reflux menstruation has so many fatal contradictions and lacks scientific proof, another mechanism of origin must be at work for the disease.

13. Is the theory of reflux menstruation correct?

No. Only circumstantial evidence exists in support of the theory of reflux menstruation as the origin of endometriosis. Circumstantial evidence is indirect evidence; it is not hard scientific proof. This theory was proposed in an era when physicians had relatively little information about or clinical experience with endometriosis, and there is no reason to think that anyone at that time would have been able to arrive at the exactly correct theory of origin of endometriosis.

The only possible way to prove that reflux menstruation is the origin of endometriosis is to find microscopic evidence of the two missing steps: (1) attachment of endometrial fragments to pelvic surfaces and (2) proliferation and invasion of these fragments into the pelvic surfaces. Supporters of reflux menstruation claim that it is very common, but evidence is lacking to prove this point. In fact, the continuing lack of what should be easily obtainable evidence is taken as an indication that the theory of reflux menstruation as the origin of endometriosis must be wrong.

Embryologically patterned metaplasia (EPM)

The theory of origin of endometriosis that fits best with existing evidence.

The myriad manifestations and differences of endometriosis from the endometrium lining the inside of the uterus arise from the plasticity of the embryo.

Gene

A segment of DNA carrying a code that directs a particular action to be taken by a cell.

14. What is the origin of endometriosis?

Since the collapse of Sampson's theory of origin, the next best candidate theory relates to **embryologically patterned metaplasia (EPM)** and cell rests.

At the moment of an individual's conception, several genetically based developmental "cards" are dealt. The first card is whether that person will develop endometriosis in the future. The second card ordains the pattern of distribution of disease in the body. The third card determines how biologically active the disease will be in each anatomical area of occurrence: even in the same pelvis, one area of disease may look rather innocuous, while another area may look florid and enraged.

The cards dealt to any particular woman are a result of a variety of factors present at the moment of conception, including genetic factors, environmental factors, and chance. As a consequence, some early embryonic cells carry genetic tags that act either alone or in concert with other **genes** to produce endometriosis. The eventual result of this discordant genetic concert is a disease that is brought to its initial manifestation during formation of the embryo due to a derangement of cell differentiation and migration.

During embryogenesis (formation of the embryo), cells are continually differentiating and migrating, perhaps at the behest of some directing anlage of the immune system, from the head toward the tail during formation of the pelvic organs. These cells migrate down across the back side of the cavity which will become the abdominal/pelvic cavity. Cells that carry the genetic tags for endometriosis migrate differently from normal cells. As a result, they do not reach their normal locations in the uterus, tubes and ovaries, but rather fall short of their intended targets. Like birds shot out of their migratory patterns in the sky, these cells typically come to lie across the bottom of the pelvis, although they could wind up anywhere in the body depending on the degree of derangement of the genetic tags. Some of these cells may be deposits of actual endometriosis, whereas others may embed themselves in tracts of tissue that will change into endometriosis during teenage years as a result of metaplasia (when one type of tissue changes into another type of tissue).

The fetal immune system may play a role in the differentiation and migration of cells during organogenesis, since cells must have some way to communicate "like" from "not like"

When the ovaries begin producing estrogen around the time of onset of menstruation, tracts of substrate of tissue begin to change into endometriosis, while if actual deposits of endometriosis were laid down, they may be stimulated to cause painful symptoms. Endometriosis continues to form from the embryologically patterned tissue tracts during the teenage years. By a woman's mid-twenties, most of the endometriosis that will ever form in her body is already present. Some of the substrate tissue may continue to change until the woman reaches her mid-thirties, creating the fibrous muscular tissue that sometimes surrounds deeply inva-sive endometriosis. Tracts of susceptible substrate tissue may be laid down in areaas far away from the pelvis, including the abdominal wall, diaphragm, or bowel.

15. Where does endometriosis most commonly occur in the pelvis?

Peritoneum

The thin, shiny, trans-parent lining of the abdomen and pelvis.

Cul-de-sac

The bottom of the pelvis. It is the most common site of occurrence of endometriosis.

The pelvic and abdominal cavities form one contiguous space and are lined by the **peritoneum**, a rather transpar-ent lining that is about the thickness of plastic kitchen wrap. Endometriosis occurs most commonly within the peritoneum, with deeper invasion possible. Among the anatomical regions of the pelvis, the **cul-de-sac** is the most common site of its occurrence; it is located at the very bottom of the pelvis, behind the uterus and in front of the rectum (**Figure 1**). The uterosacral ligaments and pelvic sidewalls are next in frequency of involvement. The ovaries are occasionally involved; when they are, the patient is more likely to have more extensive pelvic and intestinal endometriosis than do patients without ovarian disease.

16. Does endometriosis ever involve the intestines?

Ileum

The second half of the small intestine.

Cecum

The beginning of the ascending colon, located on the lower right side of the abdomen. The appendix is attached to the cecum.

Yes. The rectosigmoid colon is the most commonly involved intestinal site, followed by the end of the **ileum** (the small intestine), the **cecum** (the first part of the ascending colon on the right side of the body), and the appendix. Endometriosis of the first part of the small intestine and transverse colon is extremely rare, and this type of endometriosis is typically only superficial when it occurs.

17. Does endometriosis spread in the pelvis like dandelions over time?

No. Members of older age groups do not have more pelvic areas of involvement than members of younger age groups. Also, the surface area of pelvic involvement in older age groups is not greater than in younger age groups. Finally, when the extent of endometriosis is measured by the relatively imprecise classification system of the American Society of Reproductive Medicine, members of older age groups don't have higher-stage disease on average than members of younger age groups. This positionally static nature of endometriosis is a direct result of embryologically patterned metaplasia.

If a disease spreads in the body over time, older age groups should have more disease, as occurs with obesity or facial wrinkles. Older age groups don't have more endometriosis than younger age groups.

18. How is endometriosis staged?

The American Society of Reproductive Medicine (formerly the American Fertility Society) has a staging system that has been in use for more than 20 years. This system awards points for endometriosis as well as adhesions.

19. Is the staging system accurate and helpful?

No. Most of the points score for adhesions rather than endometriosis. The staging system does not allow precise measurement of the extent of disease or its location. The ovaries are awarded most of the endometriosis points even though they are not the most frequently involved pelvic structures. In addition, endometriosis of the intestines and diaphragm is not included in this scoring system.

The staging system for classifying endometriosis has millions of possible combinations, resulting in more possible point combinations than can be used.

For an individual patient, the classification worksheet contains 14 separate fields, each with four possible point choices, and 1 field with three point choices. This means there are more than 800 million possible combinations in which points could be scored by a single patient, but the maximum number of points allowed by the system for a single patient is 178. There are enough possible combinations of points that every woman on the face of the earth with endometriosis could be assigned a unique combination of points, but a single point total could represent millions of possible separate combinations of points. For this reason, comparing patients with the same point total can be like comparing apples to oil wells.

Because of these problems, researchers studying endometriosis have been forced to use other ways of measuring the extent of disease, such as pelvic mapping systems that identify individual anatomical regions of pelvic involvement.

20. What's the difference between deep and superficial endometriosis?

Superficial endometriosis extends less than 5 mm below the visible pelvic surface. It is usually easy to determine because the transparent peritoneum in which it rests can be pulled during surgery and it will slide across underlying blood vessels and other structures, much like pulling a shirt sleeve across the arm underneath it.

By contrast, **deep endometriosis** extends 5 mm or more beneath the visible pelvic surface. This is a somewhat arbitrary dividing line, however, and most surgeons do not use a depth gauge to measure how invasive endometriosis is. Deep disease causes the peritoneum to

Superficial endometriosis

Endometriosis that extends less than 5 mm beneath the visible pelvic surface.

Deep endometriosis

Endometriosis that extends 5 mm or more beneath the visible pelvic surface.

lose both its transparency and its ability to slide across underlying structures. Also, deep disease feels much firmer than normal tissue or superficial endometriosis.

21. What's the difference between endometriosis and pelvic pain?

The pelvis is the bony hollow contained within the pelvic bones. Pelvic pain is pain produced by any cause that occurs in the pelvis. Endometriosis is probably the most common cause of pelvic pain in women between the ages of 10 and 35, but it is not the only cause. Pelvic pain can also result from disease of the uterus, ovaries, urinary tract, intestinal tract, or musculoskeletal system.

Pelvic pain is the most common and most specific symptom of endometriosis. Endometriosis should be near the top of the list of possible causes of pelvic pain in women, but it is important to try to distinguish pain due to endometriosis from pain due to other causes, especially pain that may be coming from the uterus.

Endometriosis is the most common cause of pelvic pain in women, but not the only cause.

Leigh's story:

I had a history of endometriosis so I knew what that pain felt like. It was a burning, gnawing, stabbing pain that was really bad before a menstrual flow, but it could be present all month long. I had painful sex, too. But I had my endometriosis removed laparoscopically by excision in 2000 when I was 32, and that took care of that pain.

I did great for several years, but pain in my pelvis began to creep up on me again. But this time it felt different somehow: It didn't feel so sharp as it did before. My regular gynecologist and friends kept telling me that my endometriosis was back and that's why I was hurting again. But I wasn't so sure,

The uterus can also cause pain. Surgical treatment of endometriosis will not help pain caused by the uterus.

because I'd lived with the endometriosis pain so long that I knew what it felt like. This new pain felt more crampy, like bad menstrual cramps, and the pain radiated to my low back and down my legs. I dreaded my monthly flows.

Finally, I returned to see the doctor who took out my endometriosis before. He examined me and found that my uterus was tender but the areas of the pelvis that had been involved by endometriosis were not. He told me that he thought that my new pain was coming from my uterus, not endometriosis, and that I might need to consider having my uterus removed. Although I really didn't want to hear this, I knew in my heart that he was probably right because I'd been thinking the same thing—that it was my uterus that was the problem, not endometriosis at all.

I'm scheduled for a hysterectomy, and I'm both saddened and excited. I don't want to lose my uterus because I haven't had children. But I'm 40 and not in a relationship, and I've come to terms that I wasn't meant to have kids. I'm excited that I might get my life back, and I won't have to have my ovaries removed. Yay!

22. Can endometriosis occur outside the pelvis?

Yes. Endometriosis has been reported in the intestinal tract, urinary tract, diaphragm, muscles of the arms and legs, surgical scars on the abdomen or vagina, spinal canal, brain, lung, pelvic nerves, and the inguinal canal. This widespread distribution possible with the disease is a result of developmental abnormalities during formation of the embryo.

23. Can endometriosis occur in males?

Several case reports have described endometriosis in men, each with the same factors: elderly men with advanced prostate cancer who have received estrogen therapy to relieve painful symptoms have developed blood in the urine. Urological examination to determine the cause of this bloody urine has led to the diagnosis of endometriosis of the bladder and prostate.

The explanation for this possibility is straightforward. At 6 to 8 weeks of embryonic life, we all have within us the precursors of both the male and female reproductive systems. In genetic females, the male system is supposed to eventually wither away and disappear. In genetic males, the female system is supposed to wither away and disappear. Mother Nature is not always terribly precise, however, so this withering away process is sometimes incomplete in both males and females. If a genetic male has incomplete disappearance of the female reproductive tract during embryonic life, then tissue remnants of the female system may be left in the male pelvis. Such female tissue could respond hormonally if estrogen is given. This is another strong clue that the origin of endometriosis is in the embryo not from reflux menstruation.

Older males being treated with estrogen for prostate cancer can develop endometriosis.

PART TWO

Symptoms and Diagnosis

What are the symptoms of endometriosis?

Do I need to have surgery for diagnosis?

Are scans useful in making the diagnosis?

More . . .

24. What are the symptoms of endometriosis?

The most common symptom of endometriosis is pain. The pain is frequently geographically precise, meaning that the patient often is aware of which part of her body the pain is coming from. For example, if endometriosis is located in the cul-de-sac or uterosacral ligaments, these areas lie right at the end of the vagina and next to the rectum. Patients with disease in these areas will often complain of pain with deep penetration with intercourse or pain with bowel movements, particularly during the menstrual flow. Patients with an ovarian cyst due to endometriosis may have pain off on the side or around the flank, where pain from the ovary can radiate. Because pelvic endometriosis can occur in many separate areas, some patients have generalized pain that may not always seem localized.

Patients frequently describe pain—which is the most common symptom of endometriosis—as sharp, burning, or knifelike. The pain can occur away from the menstrual flow.

A patient's description of endometriosis pain frequently includes terms like "sharp," "knifelike," "stabbing," "like shards of glass," or other adjectives that convey a type of pain that can come on suddenly and quite noticeably. Some patients may clench their fist and make a stabbing motion toward their pelvis as they describe their pain. If an endometrioma cyst of the ovary breaks and the bloody fluid leaks out, patients may have a very severe episode of pain that peaks quickly, then subsides over the course of several days as the fluid is reabsorbed.

Endometriosis may be present but cause no pain, or it may cause mild pain that some patients may interpret as normal. If these patients have pelvic surgery for another reason, such as a new ovarian cyst causing pain, removal of endometriosis can produce pain relief.

25. How does endometriosis cause infertility?

Endometriosis is not the only cause of infertility, but it can reduce fertility is several ways. Women with endometriosis may not ovulate as well as women without the disease. Surgical removal of endometriosis may not improve ovulation even if it improves pain symptoms.

Endometriosis produces chemicals that can inflame the pelvis. The body can produce extra fluid in the pelvis as a result, similar to the fluid produced after an ankle sprain, which causes the ankle joint to swell up. This fluid contains inflammatory molecules that are produced as a normal part of the body's reaction to injury or inflammation. These molecules may damage the egg, which is bathed in these chemicals after ovulation. Also, these chemicals can be picked up by the fallopian tubes and travel down the tubes and damage any sperm that are swimming toward the end of the fallopian tube. Such damage to either the egg or the sperm may interfere with normal fertilization. Women with endometriosis who become pregnant don't have a higher chance of carrying babies with birth defects, however, so there does not appear to be any damage to the DNA of the sperm or the egg.

The fallopian tubes of women with endometriosis don't appear to have the same muscle tone as the fallopian tubes of women without endometriosis. This lack of muscle tone may interfere with the ability of the tube to "swallow" a fertilized egg toward the uterus. Women with endometriosis who conceive don't seem to have a higher chance of a tubal pregnancy, however.

Endometriosis may interfere with fertilization of the egg. Women with endometriosis may have more problems with ovulation, transport of the fertilized egg down the fallopian tube, and implantation of the embryo in the uterine lining.

The endometrium lining the uterus in women with endometriosis has certain differences compared with the endometrium in women without endometriosis. These changes may interfere with the ability of the developing embryo to implant into the uterine lining.

Women with endometriosis often have painful sexual intercourse, so they may avoid sex. This, in turn, can reduce their chance of conception.

26. At what age do symptoms start, and when is endometriosis suspected?

Women with endometriosis frequently state that they have severe pelvic pain prior to or along with their first menstrual flow. This pain may be misinterpreted by friends, family, and members of the medical profession as "just cramps" or as "part of being a woman." A young woman who has never had a menstrual flow would not know the difference between uterine cramping or pain due to endometriosis, which sets the stage for years of suffering because the pain is thought to be a normal process. It is common for women who reports such pain to be belittled by others, because they cannot feel the misery the patient is going through. The patient may be told that "It can't be that bad" or "I had cramps, too, but I just learned to live with it." The end result of this disconnect is that many women with endometriosis are told, "It's all in your head."

Severe pelvic pain keeping a teen from school needs to be evaluated by a gynecologist for the possibility of endometriosis.

As time goes by, various other layers of pain may be added. For example, when sexual activity begins, painful intercourse may occur. At this point, the woman may be told that she's "uncomfortable with being a woman." Painful bowel movements may eventually occur, with "more fiber in the diet" being recommended. If the young woman misses school or work because of pain, she may be accused of "making it all up" or trying to avoid exams or unpleasant surroundings.

When the patient goes to the doctor because of pain, sexually transmitted disease (STD) is often diagnosed, even when the patient is a virgin and has negative tests. Antibiotics may be given to treat presumed pelvic inflammatory disease. Antibiotics may be repeated when the patient seems to have reacquired an STD the following month. When pain pills are used to treat the symptom of pain, requests by the patient for refills are often deemed "drug-seeking behavior." When the patient sees other physicians to try to get an answer, she may be accused of "doctor shopping."

For these reasons, the delay in diagnosis of endometriosis is typically between 8 and 11 years.

Mary's story:

I am so mad. I wasted so much time, and I'm worried that I've damaged my chances of getting pregnant. No one would listen to me when I was hurting. Everyone kept telling me that I was making it up and that things couldn't be as bad as I was letting on. But I was feeling the pain—they weren't. I was misdiagnosed with so many crazy things over the years. Venereal disease, even though I hadn't had sex yet. Adhesions due to the venereal disease. Ovarian cysts, even though all the ultrasounds ever showed was some fluid in my pelvis. They never found a cyst on ultrasound, even days before they would diagnose a ruptured cyst. I had all kinds of tests that I didn't need, including colonoscopy, bladder examinations, MRI and CT scans, blood tests. They were all normal. When I would ask for something to relieve the pain, I felt guilty because they told me that I was getting addicted and seeking narcotics like I was a drug addict.

After the onset of painful symptoms, the typical delay in diagnosis of endometriosis is almost 10 years. Unfortunately, pelvic pain in women is often not taken seriously by society.

This went on from the age of 12 to the age of 20. I was finally diagnosed with endometriosis then. I felt relieved that there really was something going on that could explain the pain, since I'd been thinking that it was all in my head. Now that I have a name for what's going on, it helps me deal with it a little better, but the pain still hurts and I'm mad for how long it took to get a correct diagnosis. Sometimes I think no one is listening to me.

27. What are the symptoms of intestinal endometriosis?

Intestinal endometriosis begins on the surface of the bowel and may invade into the muscle layer. It rarely goes all the way through the bowel wall. The recto-sigmoid colon is the bowel area that is most commonly involved, followed by the terminal ileum (the part of the small bowel near its junction with the large bowel), the appendix, and the cecum (the beginning of the ascending colon). Among women with intestinal involvement, 29% have more than one intestinal area involved. Intestinal endometriosis may cause no symptoms if it is superficial on the bowel surface. It causes symptoms when it invades the muscular layer of the bowel, resulting in distortion of the bowel wall.

The symptoms of bowel obstruction include nausea and vomiting after eating, abdominal bloating, intestinal cramping, intestinal pain, right lower quadrant pain, and weight loss.

The symptoms of intestinal endometriosis depend on two issues: (1) the degree of distortion of the bowel wall and (2) the site of intestinal involvement. The more severe the invasion, the more bowel wall distortion that occurs, and the more severe the symptoms tend to be. In the large bowel, the distortion tends to be spherical. In the small bowel, the muscular layer is thinner, and the distortion tends to be more linear along the length of the bowel involved. In either the large or small bowel, this distortion can cause the bowel to fold back on itself,

Bowel obstruction by endometriosis is usually partial. The more severe the obstruction, the more severe the symptoms may be.

like an arm bending at the elbow. Intestinal contents can have difficulty passing through such a tight bend, and symptoms of bowel obstruction may occur. Because the diameter of the small bowel is smaller than the diameter of the large bowel, symptoms of bowel obstruction are more common when severe distortion is present in the small intestine.

Although cyclic rectal bleeding occurring simultaneously with the menstrual flow is uncommon in women with intestinal endometriosis, when such a bleeding pattern is present, it often means that the endometriosis has penetrated the full thickness of the bowel wall.

Symptoms of rectal endometriosis include rectal pain with bowel movements all month long, rectal pain with passing gas, and rectal pain with sitting. The nodule in the bowel wall results in a sense of rectal fullness, so some patients will have a sense of incomplete bowel emptying after bowel movements. Symptoms of sigmoid endometriosis include left lower quadrant pain prior to bowel movements and sometimes a sense of constipation.

Symptoms of endometriosis of the ileum include right lower quadrant pain and symptoms of partial bowel obstruction. Complete bowel obstruction is rare; when it occurs, patients are violently ill.

When the appendix is involved by endometriosis, the patient may not have any symptoms. Occasionally, mild right lower quadrant pain may be present. Endometriosis of the appendix does not cause symptoms resembling acute appendicitis.

Because of the relatively large diameter of the cecum, endometriosis in this area usually causes no symptoms.

Because of its smaller diameter, the small intestine is more easily obstructed than the large intestine. The terminal ileum is the bowel area that is most commonly obstructed.

Superficial or slightly invasive endometriosis of the cul-de-sac can cause painful bowel movements during the menstrual flow. Deeply invasive endometriosis with rectal involvement can produce painful bowel movements all month long.

Jennifer's story:

*They thought that I had an eating disorder. I was both-
ered by nausea, vomiting, and weight loss. If I tried to take
anything by mouth other than liquids, my symptoms would
occur. This had been worsening for several months, and I'd
dropped from 125 pounds to 85 pounds. I had all kinds of
tests done, including barium studies and colonoscopy. They
couldn't figure out what was going on, so that's why they
thought I had bulimia or anorexia, even though I was in
my mid-thirties. I thought younger women usually had
those things.*

*I continued to lose weight and had been in a hospital in
a large city. I was getting very upset and worried because
there seemed to be no answer and no treatment, and I was
worried I was going to die. I'm married and I'd wanted to
have children, not become a poster child for whatever weird
disease was killing me. I became very depressed, which rein-
forced the doctors' opinion that this was a psychological issue
and that I wanted attention.*

*Finally, my GI doctor called an endometriosis surgeon who
lived in a city several hours away. The surgeon told my doctor
over the phone that he thought I had endometriosis obstructing my small bowel. Yeah, right, I thought. Why hadn't they
found it then? They transferred me to the other hospital,
and I had surgery the next day. They found extensive endometriosis of the pelvis and an obstructing nodule of my small
intestine. I had another partially obstructing nodule of my
sigmoid colon. I had all my pelvic endometriosis removed
and two segmental bowel resections done laparoscopically
through really tiny incisions. I had an uneventful recovery.
I was too scared to hope that this would work, since nothing
in the big city had worked.*

I finally believed it worked when my pain was completely gone and I could eat whatever I wanted when I got home. I regained my weight, got pregnant, and now have a beautiful baby boy. I shake my head when I think that I almost died.

28. What are the symptoms of endometriosis of the urinary tract?

Endometriosis can affect the bladder and the **ureters** (the hollow, muscular tubes carrying urine from the kidneys down to the bladder). Superficial disease of the bladder usually causes no symptoms. Similar to intestinal endometriosis, when bladder endometriosis begins to invade the bladder muscle, symptoms may occur. Patients with deeply invasive bladder disease often complain of bladder pain as the bladder empties. Endometriosis of the bladder usually doesn't penetrate all the way through the bladder wall, so blood in the urine is uncommon.

Endometriosis affecting a ureter is always an extension of invasive disease from an adjacent uterosacral ligament. Most commonly, the ureter is surrounded by fibrotic **scar tissue**, which can sometimes constrict the ureter. Rarely will endometriosis invade the muscular wall of the ureter. When it does, blood may be visible in the urine or found on a dipstick test.

When the ureter is constricted, urine can back up into the kidney, which causes severe, deep flank pain (**Figure 4**). The constriction (and the pain) may be worse during a menstrual flow because of tissue swelling around the ureter. Occasionally a ureter will become constricted so slowly that it does not produce any kidney symptoms. In these cases, patients may lose the function of a kidney as a result of long-standing "silent" constriction of the ureter.

Ureter

A hollow, muscular tube about the diameter of a pencil that drains urine from a kidney down into the bladder.

Scar tissue

Fibrous tissue that forms as a result of healing of an injury or inflammation in the body.

If the ureter is blocked by stricture related to invasion of the ureter, the kidney on that side can lose its function silently and permanently.

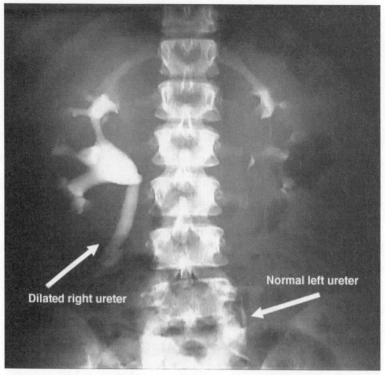

Figure 4 Intravenous pyelogram x-ray showing massive dilation of right ureter because it is obstructed by endometriosis down near the bladder.

Amniocentesis is when a needle is inserted through a pregnant woman's abdominal wall into the uterus in order to withdraw amniotic fluid. Endometriosis has been reported in a needle tract from amniocentesis.

29. What are the symptoms of endometriosis in a surgical scar?

Endometriosis can be found in surgical scars such as an episiotomy incision (a cut to enlarge the vaginal opening during delivery of a baby) or an abdominal incision, most commonly following a cesarean section. Months or years later, a painful lump that swells during the menstrual flow may appear.

30. What are the symptoms of endometriosis of the diaphragm?

The diaphragm is the breathing muscle separating the abdominal cavity from the chest cavity. It is only about 0.25 inch thick. Endometriosis involves the right diaphragm much more commonly than the left diaphragm. When diaphragmatic endometriosis causes symptoms, it has always invaded the full thickness of the diaphragm. Symptoms of diaphragmatic endometriosis include chest and shoulder pain on the involved side. The pain may worsen prior to and during the menstrual flow. Sometimes the pain may extend up the side of the neck or down the arm. In some cases, the pain may be so severe that it can be difficult to take a breath. Occasionally, the patient must sleep upright.

31. How does endometriosis cause painful intercourse?

The most common pelvic site involved by endometriosis is the cul-de-sac, which is located just on the other side of the end of the vagina. The vagina is only about 0.25 inch thick, so during intercourse, the penis can hit the area involved by endometriosis fairly directly, causing pain—a condition known as **dyspareunia**.

Dyspareunia

Painful sexual intercourse.

32. Is there a blood test for endometriosis?

There is no reliable blood test for endometriosis. The CA-125 level is sometimes obtained, but will be normal in most patients and elevated in only a fraction of patients with deeply invasive disease. The CA-125 level can also be elevated in women with uterine fibroids, adenomyosis of the uterus, pelvic adhesions, and ovarian cancer, and in some women with no apparent disease , and other diseases that provoke an inflammatory response. A blood test would be useful in the future if a truly effective form of medical treatment for endometriosis is found.

The white blood count and erythrocyte sedimentation rate are nonspecific measures of inflammation or infection in the body; these measures increase in conditions such as appendicitis, kidney infection, and other diseases that provoke an autoimmune response. Although the pain caused by endometriosis can be severe, the results of these two tests are usually in the normal range.

33. What does the doctor look for during a pelvic examination?

A simple pelvic examination can give a good idea of whether endometriosis is present.

A pelvic examination has two parts: the speculum exam and the manual exam. The speculum can be used for more than just taking a Pap smear. In some women with rectal nodules of endometriosis or nodules of the uterosacral ligaments, endometriosis invades the vagina just behind the cervix. This area can be seen if the speculum is tilted toward the rear, although not all gynecologists perform this simple maneuver. This manifestation of endometriosis represents the only instance when endometriosis can be diagnosed with 100% accuracy without surgery.

Endometrioma

An ovarian cyst caused by endometriosis.

Because most women with endometriosis will not have vaginal involvement, the manual part of the pelvic exam is the most important component in making a diagnosis. Occasionally, if a patient has an ovarian cyst caused by endometriosis (an **endometrioma**), the doctor may be able to feel enlargement of the ovary, although this enlargement could also be due to many other disease processes besides endometriosis. Doctors can't tell the difference between causes of ovarian enlargement by manual exam alone. Occasionally a transvaginal ultrasound may give a little more information, but not all doctors perform these exams in their offices.

The biggest payoff during pelvic exam comes during palpation of the cul-de-sac and uterosacral ligaments. These areas are easily reached if the doctor's fingers are long enough. Normally, these areas should not be tender when gently palpated or stroked. When endometriosis is present, the patient will usually grimace her face in pain or move up on the exam table away from the doctor. If painful lumps are found in the cul-de-sac or uterosacral ligaments, their presence increases the likelihood of endometriosis to more than 95%.

Lori's story:

During the pelvic exam, the doctor kept hitting an area that hurt. I told her that the exam was causing pain just like what I had at home. She looked cross at me and told me in a stern voice, "Relax! An exam should not hurt that much. Don't be such a baby." I didn't get to talk with her afterward, because she was called to deliver a baby. I talked with her nurse, who said that many women don't like pelvic exams, and I shouldn't feel too bad for reacting the way I did. They tried to make it sound like I could control myself when it was painful. I'd like to see them try to hold their hand over a flame. When it hurts, you just can't help it.

34. How is endometriosis diagnosed?

A diagnosis may be either a **differential diagnosis** or a definitive diagnosis. A differential diagnosis is a list of possible diagnoses based on the history, physical exam, and any tests. A differential diagnosis represents the doctor's best guess about what might be going on. In

Differential diagnosis

A list of possible diagnoses based on the patient's history, physical exam and other tests; the doctor's best guess.

addition to endometriosis, a typical differential diagnosis list for pelvic pain in women would include less common conditions such as ruptured ovarian cysts, adhesions, or pelvic infections caused by a sexually transmitted disease. Because evidence of endometriosis doesn't always appear on scans and other tests, some patients may be told that they have nothing wrong with them because "all their tests are normal."

Definitive diagnosis

A diagnosis that has been absolutely confirmed.

A **definitive diagnosis** means the diagnosis is absolutely confirmed. Endometriosis can be absolutely confirmed either by visualizing it or preferably by biopsy and examination through a microscope. In more than 99% of patients with endometriosis, it is necessary to perform surgery to make a definitive diagnosis.

35. What is laparoscopy?

Laparoscope

A tube that is typically 5–10 mm in diameter, through which a physician can visualize internal organs and pass instruments to perform surgery.

A **laparoscope** is a tube which is typically between 5 mm and 10 mm in diameter. Fiber-optic bundles are contained within the tube. One set of bundles transmits light to the end of the laparoscope, and another set of bundles transmits the view from the end of the laparoscope back up to an eyepiece. Laparoscopy has been in use since the 1930's. Room air pumped into the patient by a foot pump was used in those days to distend the abdomen.

Laparoscopy

The surgical use of a laparoscope to diagnose or treat disease.

Laparoscopy (Figure 5) is the action of viewing the contents of the abdominal or pelvic cavity with a laparoscope. Carbon dioxide gas is pumped into the abdominal cavity to create a bubble with a volume of about 3 liters. The viewing tip of the laparoscope is placed within this bubble, with the panorama of the intestines and pelvic organs spread out across the bottom of the bubble.

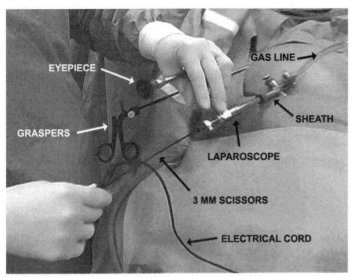

Figure 5 A 10-mm diameter operating laparoscope is inserted through a metal sheath in the umbilicus.

Otherwise, it would be impossible to visualize anything, like putting the tip of the laparoscope under a pillow or into a bowl of cooked spaghetti.

Some laparoscopes contain an operating channel that spans the length of the instrument, so a surgical tool such as scissors can be passed into the abdomen to assist in performing surgery. To facilitate visualization and to perform surgery, other small-diameter tools are inserted through separate tiny incisions.

In diagnostic laparoscopy, the laparoscope is used only to view the contents of the **peritoneal cavity** and no surgery is performed. Operative laparoscopy involves performing surgery through the laparoscope. In gynecological surgery, there would seldom be a reason to perform only a diagnostic laparoscopy.

Generations of gynecologists have been taught that the characteristic visual appearance of endometriosis looked like a "black powder-burn." This presentation is actually far less common than originally thought, which contributes to the confusion surrounding this disease.

Peritoneal cavity

The internal bodily cavity lined by the peritoneum. This cavity contains the intestines, liver, spleen, and female pelvic organs.

Laparotomy

Opening the abdominal cavity with an incision made with a scalpel.

The suffix -otomy means to cut something open.

In **laparotomy**, a scalpel is used to make a large incision in the abdominal wall through which surgery can be done. Virtually any surgery that can be done by laparotomy can be performed laparoscopically with less trauma, less pain, and less recovery time.

36. What does endometriosis look like at surgery?

Every intellectual and therapeutic process involving endometriosis begins with a surgeon identifying disease in the pelvis, so the visual appearance of endometriosis is quite important.

Endometriosis involving the peritoneum, which lines the pelvic cavity, can have many different visual appearances. In young women, it may take the form of a clear lesion, looking almost like dewdrops on a plant. It can also look like the translucent grains in tapioca pudding (**Figure 6**). The glandular elements of endometriosis sometimes secrete a substance (which has not been analyzed as yet) that seems able to destabilize surrounding capillaries, causing them to bleed. Also secreted is a substance that, in some patients, can invite the growth of small new blood vessels into the area.

Bleeding associated with endometriosis is due to fragility of capillaries nearby the endometriosis, not from the endometriosis itself.

As the inflammatory effects of the disease add up, scar tissue can begin to cover the lesion, giving it a whitish or yellowish appearance and hiding the actual lesions of endometriosis. Some surgeons mistakenly call this "burned out" disease, but is actually highly biologically active "burned in" disease.

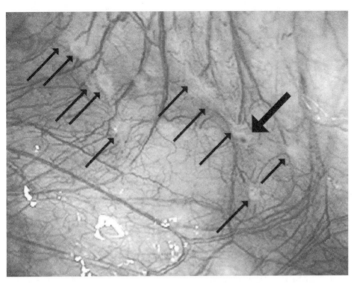

Figure 6 Subtle "tapioca" lesions of endometriosis (thin arrows) in a young woman. Only one of the lesions has any bleeding associated with it (thick arrow). Two lesions have not been marked with arrows. Can you find them?

As more capillary bleeding adjacent to endometriosis occurs, the blood gets trapped under the scar tissue and turns darker. This produces a blackish discoloration amid the scarring—the classic "black powderburn" lesion seen in older women. This "black powderburn" lesion is the only visual appearance that many doctors have been trained to look for.

Teenagers can have very subtle disease that can be easily missed.

Not all lesions of endometriosis go through this evolution of visual appearance, however. Depending on the degree of biological activity imparted at the moment of conception, some lesions may remain innocuous in appearance, although lesions of any appearance can still cause pain and contribute to infertility. In some patients, muscle tissue begins to form around the endometriosis by a process called **metaplasia**. The resulting lumps or nodules are found primarily in the uterosacral ligaments, the wall of the bladder, and the wall of the rectum.

Fibromuscular metaplasia

The formation of muscle tissue around an area of endometriosis.

37

The age-related change in the color of endometriosis can have surprising effects. If a surgeon overlooks some subtle disease in a teenager but another surgeon finds more obvious disease in the same patient several years later, the impression would be that new disease had appeared. This would give false support to the theory of reflux menstruation because someone could say, "See? This patient didn't have any disease at her first laparoscopy but had disease at her second surgery, which must prove Sampson's theory of reflux menstruation."

Not every visual abnormality found on the peritoneum is necessarily endometriosis. Carbon left behind by previous **laser** vaporization can look black and might be confused as endometriosis. Scarring from previous surgery may be misinterpreted as whitish endometriosis. Chronic inflammation and microcalcifications may also be misidentified visually as endometriosis.

Ovarian endometriosis can look like red spots on the white surface of the ovary, or it can form a cyst called an endometrioma that is filled with dark bloody fluid. When the bloody fluid is old and stagnant, it thickens and resembles chocolate sauce, so the term "chocolate cyst" is sometimes used to describe this finding. **Corpus luteum cysts** are normal ovarian cysts that form after ovulation each month. They sometimes bleed internally, and reactive scar tissue may form around them, which can make them look exactly like an endometrioma cyst.

Endometriosis of the intestinal tract usually lacks significant surrounding bleeding, so the surgeon must look for innocuous flat colorless or grayish lesions. When intestinal endometriosis is more florid, a golf-ball size nodule with scarring may be present, yet little or no adjacent bleeding may occur.

Laser

Acronym for "light amplification of stimulated emission radiation." In medical use, refers to a high-powered, focused beam of light used to perform surgery.

Corpus luteum cyst

A cyst formed by the ovary every month at the site of ovulation. Corpus luteum cysts can look just like endometrioma cysts on ultrasound or at surgery, but pathological examination under a microscope can tell the difference.

When the rectum has a nodule of endometriosis, it sometimes will scar forward to the back of the uterus, resulting in **obliteration of the cul-de-sac**. This condition represents invasive endometriosis of the underlying uterosacral ligaments, the cul-de-sac, the rear of the cervix, and usually the front wall of the rectum. Unfortunately, many surgeons looking at this most severe visual manifestation of endometriosis view it as primarily a problem of scar tissue formation rather than as the presence of underlying biologically active disease, which remains hidden beneath what can sometimes seem a rather bland surface appearance.

Endometriosis of the left diaphragm can usually be seen with a laparoscope inserted through the umbilicus because the left lobe of the liver is small and doesn't hide the left diaphragm. Endometriosis of the right diaphragm is much more common than left-sided disease, but the right lobe of the liver is very large and can hide symptomatic endometriosis. All the surgeon might see would be small "sentinel" lesions on the front side of the diaphragm. To see the back side of the diaphragm clearly, it is frequently necessary to put a small-diameter laparoscope under the edge of the right rib cage so that the laparoscope can pass over the liver and view the back part of the diaphragm directly.

Obliteration of the cul-de-sac

The rectum scars forward to the rear of the cervix so the cul-de-sac can't be seen. This signifies invasive endometriosis of the underlying uterosacral ligaments, the cul-de-sac, the rear of the cervix, and usually the front wall of the rectum.

37. Is some endometriosis "invisible" at surgery?

Not really. Endometriosis or changes caused by it are always visible when they are present. Even a small lesion of endometriosis is larger than the diameter of a human hair. Endometrioisis should be readily visible during laparoscopy because the laparoscope gives a magnified

Even small endometriosis lesions are larger across than the diameter of a human hair.

view of the details of the pelvic surface. If a doctor expects endometriosis to look like a "black powderburn" lesion, then lesions of other colors may go unnoticed.

Sometimes endometriosis can be buried under scar tissue, in which case the doctor can't actually see the endometriosis. Although the endometriosis may be "invisible" beneath all of the surrounding tissue, the surface changes over it are not. These abnormalities should draw the attention of a knowledgeable surgeon, who should suspect that underlying endometriosis exists.

Although rare reports have outlined deposits of endometriosis found under normal peritoneum, the concept that visually normal peritoneum frequently harbors "invisible" microscopic endometriosis is false and unscientific. Researchers have looked for this evidence and have never found it. Medicine should be based on science, not firmly held beliefs.

38. Do I need to have surgery for diagnosis?

Usually yes. One manifestation of endometriosis that can be diagnosed without surgery is when the rear wall of the vagina is involved by the disease. This condition can be seen in the doctor's office with a speculum. Women with this finding usually have very extensive pelvic and frequently intestinal involvement. Endometriosis of the belly button can also be seen without surgery.

39. Are scans helpful in making the diagnosis?

Sometimes. Most cases of endometriosis exist as flat lesions of various colors that cannot be detected by any scan. For something to show up on ultrasound, computerized tomography (CT), or magnetic resonance imaging (MRI)—the three most common types of imaging studies—it usually must have sufficient three-dimensional volume, usually being about the size of a pea or larger. For example, a sunburn of the skin has a large length and a large width, but because it is flat, it won't show up on any scan.

Also, for something to show up on a scan, it must be sufficiently different in density from the tissue surrounding it to stand out in contrast. For example, a marble suspended in Jello would readily show up on any scan: The marble is large enough and different enough from the surrounding "tissue" that it can be found easily. Nodular endometriosis can be woody and fibrotic, which is different from normal tissue. For this reason, some large nodules associated with endometriosis will show up on scans. However, by the time a nodule shows up on a scan, the physician should already be suspicious of the existence of such a finding based on the patient's history of significant pain and a pelvic examination where tender nodularity is found.

Another form of endometriosis that can be found by scans is an endometrioma cyst of the ovary. These cysts have the size and the density difference from surrounding tissue needed to show up well on imaging studies, although the ultrasonographer can't be certain what type of cyst has been found. Corpus luteum cysts caused by ovulation can look identical to endometrioma cysts on ultrasound.

Surgery is more accurate than any scan for diagnosing endometriosis.

40. Can medicines be used to diagnose endometriosis?

Improvement of pain with medical therapy can't be used as an indication of whether the patient has endometriosis.

No, although the manufacturer of leuprolide acetate would have doctors believe this in an effort to sell more product. Leuprolide works by putting the ovaries to sleep temporarily, with the result that the woman's estrogen level drops markedly, sending her into something resembling the menopausal state. The woman's menstrual flow frequently stops as a result. The manufacturer of this medication has convinced doctors that if a patient's pain improves while on the medication, then her pain must be due to endometriosis.

The problem with this notion is that many painful conditions might be less painful if the estrogen level in the body is lower. These conditions include adenomyosis of the uterus, fibroid tumors of the uterus, ovulation pain, painful menstrual cramps, and menstrual migraine headaches. So, reduction or elimination of pain with use of leuprolide acetate does not help differentiate among these causes of pain.

41. How does endometriosis cause pain?

The glandular elements of endometriosis secrete a substance that leaches directly into surrounding tissue, irritating nerves, destabilizing capillaries, and resulting in scar tissue.

Endometriosis is composed of glandular tissue surrounded by tissue called stroma. All glandular tissues secrete substances. For example, sweat glands secrete sweat; saliva glands secrete saliva. We don't know exactly what the glands involved in endometriosis secrete, but it is probably different from what the endometrial glands of the uterine lining secrete. This substance leaks out into surrounding tissue and can be very irritating. It can be likened to a mild acid in its actions (the actual secretions themselves may not actually be acidic, but the analogy works for this discussion). These secretions can destabilize adjacent capillaries, causing them to bleed, which may be part of the pain that women with endometriosis experience. Of course, many endometriosis lesions are not associated with any bleeding at all, so the secretions themselves must have the ability to irritate tiny nerves in the peritoneal lining and the surrounding tissues. Imagine lemon juice getting into a paper cut—it wouldn't take much to cause pain.

If scar tissue has formed in response to endometriosis, the scar tissue can pull on structures like a rope, which can cause pain. Most women with endometriosis do not have a lot of scar tissue, though.

42. Does endometriosis always cause pain?

Perhaps not. Some women with no complaint of pelvic pain may undergo surgery for a reason unrelated to endometriosis or pelvic pain, and endometriosis may be found unexpectedly. In one study of women undergoing laparoscopy for sterilization, endometriosis was found in approximately 40% of the women. Interestingly, if endometriosis is removed from "asymptomatic" women, some will report later that they realized that they were having pain, but that they thought it was normal or it never reached a bothersome level. Small amounts of endometriosis may cause lots of pain, and large amounts may cause lower levels of pain. Pain relief should be the goal of treatment, no matter how much endometriosis is present.

The degree of the patient's symptoms does not always correlate with the amount of disease.

PART THREE

Symptomatic Treatment

What is symptomatic treatment?

What are medical therapies based on?

What if medicine doesn't relieve my pain?

More . . .

43. What is symptomatic treatment?

Symptomatic treatment is directed at relieving symptoms, rather than treating the disease. When doctors or patients think of treatment of a disease, they understandably think of using a medicine to eradicate the cause of disease, such as antibiotic treatment for pneumonia or urinary tract infection. Medical therapy of endometriosis is not medical treatment in this classical sense, because there is no medicine that eradicates endometriosis. All medicines for endometriosis treat the symptoms but not the disease. Once medical therapy is finished, the patient will still have all of the disease she started with. If the patient achieved any pain relief during medical therapy, the pain begins to return in most cases within 2 weeks to 2 months.

Despite their shortcomings, medical therapies are popular with health maintenance organizations (HMOs) and capitated health plans, which make a certain number of dollars available each year for the care of a population (the subscribers to the plan). The popularity of medical therapy stems primarily from the fact that a few months of this kind of therapy is cheaper than surgery. These businesses can point to the favorable articles on medical therapy published by drug manufacturers as scientifi support for this economically based treatment plan.

Hormonal suppression of the ovaries to treat endometriosis is based on the unproven notions that pregnancy and menopause eradicate endometriosis.

44. What are medical therapies based on?

Medical therapy is based on selection bias, leaps of faith, and unsubstantiated conclusions that are based on the response of symptoms to the treatment rather than the response of the underlying disease. Its roots date back to the 1920s, before anyone knew much about all of the possible causes of infertility, such as ovulation problems, sperm problems, blocked fallopian tubes, and so on. At that time, it was assumed that normal fertility should be close to 100% among married women. When a lower fertility rate among married women with endometriosis was observed, it was assumed that endometriosis reduced fertility. While this part of the conclusion may be correct, an unsupported leap of faith was made when it was pronounced that pregnancy must protect against endometriosis. This part of the conclusion had no supporting evidence, yet has been repeated to this day.

A related observation was made in the 1920s about menopausal women. Among several women with endometriosis profiled in one study, no menopausal women were found. It was assumed, therefore, that menopause must protect against endometriosis.

Thus many modern medical therapies directed at the symptoms of endometriosis are based on observations in small groups of women, with the subsequent leaps of faith resulting in unsupported conclusions. These leaps of faith continued and worsened into the late twentieth century, because by then it was a firmly established belief that both pregnancy and menopause actually destroyed endometriosis. The proof of these twin notions would be simple: Diagnose endometriosis surgically in symptomatic women but don't treat them. Follow them through a pregnancy or after menopause, and then reoperate to see whether the disease is gone.

In fact, there is no evidence that either pregnancy or the menopause destroys endometriosis and makes it go away. Despite this lack of evidence, the main medical therapies are based on these hormonal states. Birth control pills and progesterone therapy seek to mimic the hormonal effects of pregnancy, while gonadotropin-releasing hormone (GnRH) agonists seek to mimic the hormonal effects of menopause.

Many of the guiding principles of modern therapy originated from small, exploratory studies carried out in the 1920s.

Medical cure of endometriosis has never been proved even though many patients are told that endometriosis can be cured by medicines.

Beverly's story:

I took medicines to treat my endometriosis. First I took the pill. Then I took a male-type hormone. Last I took a shot that put me into menopause. I guess the reason I took so many medicines was that none of them worked, at least not for very long.

Near the end of each round of medicine, I had another surgery to see if the endometriosis was gone—it was always there. I was told that this was the way endometriosis was treated, and that my disease should be gone, but that I had a resistant case. Each time I finished the medicine, I had about 3 weeks of less pain, but then the pain started coming back. I was told that it was because the endometriosis would always come back and that there was no good treatment.

All the medicines had side effects, and the shot was the worst. It also cost a lot of money and insurance didn't pay for it. Now I'm in pain again and I don't know if I can afford more treatment. My doctor said I might need a hysterectomy. I feel like the medicines really haven't done anything.

45. How do hormonal therapies for endometriosis work, and what are their side effects?

Most birth control pills contain both an estrogen and a progesterone-like hormone. Birth control pills work by suppressing ovulation from the ovaries, although that is not their main goal in treating endometriosis symptoms. When ovulation is suppressed, the ovaries no longer manufacture estrogen and progesterone. By shutting down the ovaries, the birth control pill replaces the cycling levels of these two ovarian hormones with a steady-state level of both estrogen and a progesterone-like hormone.

This is supposed to mimic the steady-state level of hormones during pregnancy, inducing a condition known as **pseudo-pregnancy**. However, true pregnancy has a much higher hormonal effect on the female body, with elevated levels of estrogen and especially progesterone.

All birth control pills on the market are low-dose pills, which means that the birth control pill can never approach the true hormonal effects of pregnancy. Nonetheless, birth control pills can occasionally improve symptoms of endometriosis, in part by reducing or eliminating the menstrual flow. Symptoms that are not directly related to endometriosis, such as uterine cramping with the menstrual flow, may be relieved as well. The birth control pill can be given continuously indefinitely so long as bothersome side effects don't develop. The side effects of birth control pills range from trivial to severe, including irregular bleeding, weight gain, high blood pressure, depression, mood changes, gallstones, blood clots in the legs, heart attacks, and strokes. The serious side effects are very rare. Smoking slightly increases the risks associated with birth control pills, so store clerks selling cigarettes to women should ask if they are on the pill and refuse to make sales to those women who are.

Progesterone and progesterone-like hormones called **progestins** are sometimes used alone to treat the symptoms of endometriosis. These hormones can stop ovulation and seek to mimic the high steady-state progesterone effect of pregnancy. They can be given in the form of pills or injections. Side effects of progesterone include irregular bleeding, depression and weight gain. **Intrauterine devices (IUDs)** loaded with progesterone can be inserted into the uterus as contraceptives and may decrease the menstrual flow and uterine cramps with fewer side effects on the body. Irregular bleeding may still result.

Pseudo-pregnancy

a hormonal state induced by birth control pills that somewhat mimics the hormonal state of pregnancy.

Progestins

Artificial hormones that mimic the effects of the natural hormone progesterone.

Intrauterine device (IUD)

A small plastic device, sometimes impregnated with a progestin, that is placed inside the uterus to prevent pregnancy by interfering with implantation of the embryo.

SYMPTOMATIC TREATMENT

GnRH agonists are usually given by injection and may shut the ovaries down more profoundly than the birth control pill. GnRH agonists do not have a primary hormonal effect mimicking either estrogen or progesterone, which means that many patients will have no estrogen in their body, a condition known as **pseudo-menopause**. This can lead to bothersome menopausal side effects such as hot flashes, night sweats, and vaginal dryness. Many women complain of joint aches and pains, problems with memory, weight gain, and mood swings. Some of these side effects continue long after the medicine is stopped. Loss of skeletal calcium can also occur. To combat side effects and loss of calcium, estrogen is sometimes given as "add-back" therapy to counteract the low estrogen levels seen with GnRH agonist therapy.

GnRH agonists are used only to treat symptoms of pain and can relieve estrogen-related pain from several causes besides endometriosis. These medications are not used to treat infertile women with endometriosis, because they do not improve fertility; in fact, they may actually be associated with a decrease in fertility. The reason for this decline in fertility is related to a woman's decline of fertility with advancing age. Women are most fertile between ages 15 and 25, with fertility declining progressively rapidly thereafter. By the age of 40, a woman's chance for natural conception is approximately 2%. If a woman takes a GnRH agonist for the recommended 6 months, then she will be less fertile when she stops therapy because of the natural background decline in her fertility. GnRH agonists are also expensive, with monthly costs ranging between $300 and $500. Because symptom relief occurs primarily during treatment and does not last very long when treatment is stopped, the cost of a pain-free month is more than twice the cost of a pain-free month following surgery.

Wanda's story:

I was given GnRH agonist injections for my endometriosis pain. It made the pain go away while I was taking it, but I had a lot of side effects like hot flashes, night sweats, and vaginal irritation. I now know what it's like to be in menopause. Some side effects were a little surprising. I had aches and pains in my joints and muscles. I still have some memory issues, and I gained some weight.

Danazol is an older medicine that also seeks to mimic menopause by suppressing ovarian function. It is a derivative of a male hormone, so its side-effect profile includes masculinization features such as scalp hair loss, facial hair growth, reduction in breast size, deepening of the voice, and growth of the clitoris.

46. Are newer drugs under study?

Some newer drugs under study are not hormonally based and represent a welcome departure from the past, although their efficacy remains in question.

Aromatase is an enzyme that is secreted by some endometriosis lesions. It converts a precursor molecule in the bloodstream into estrogen. In this way, endometriosis is able to manufacture its own estrogen even if the ovaries have been removed. This process may be one reason why postmenopausal women occasionally have symptomatic endometriosis. Aromatase inhibitors block the action of aromatase, so that endometriosis lesions producing aromatase cannot manufacture estrogen. This blockade can reduce endometriosis symptoms, although there is no evidence that it eradicates the actual endometriosis. How long the effect lasts after treatment stops and what percentage of women will be helped by this therapy are issues that remain under study.

Endometriosis can produce its own estrogen supply using the aromatase enzyme.

Angiogenesis

Growth of new blood vessels (*angio-* means "blood").

Growth of new blood vessels (**angiogenesis**) is part of the normal inflammatory response to injury. Endometriosis can be associated with the growth of new blood vessels into the areas involved by endometriosis. By stopping the growth of these new blood vessels, researchers hope to influence the activity and development of endometriosis. Medicines that block the growth of new blood vessels are currently under study.

Unfortunately, there are several problems with this approach. Researchers have started with the hypothesis that endometriosis needs new blood vessel growth to exist. This assumption ignores the fact that endometriosis was present before the growth of the blood vessels. Also, not all lesions of endometriosis are associated with the growth of new blood vessels, which means there are sometimes no new vessels to inhibit. This lack of blood vessel growth is observed in both superficial peritoneal lesions and the middle of large nodules, where almost no blood vessels are visible. Also, the idea of stopping angiogenesis might have detrimental effects elsewhere in the body: New vessel growth may be required for normal wound healing in other parts of the body, so will inhibiting new vessel growth be associated with some severe disturbance of wound healing and tissue repair? Finally, the efficacy in treating symptomatic patients needs to be defined.

47. What if medicine doesn't relieve my pain?

There are only three options for treating disease: do nothing, treat the condition with medicine, or treat the condition with surgery. If medical therapy of symptoms proves ineffective, a final form of medical management of symptoms can be used called pain management. **Pain management centers** are staffed by physicians who prescribe medicines such as narcotics, antidepressants, and neuromodulators (medicines that affect the way nerves transmit pain signals) in an attempt to relieve their patients' symptoms. Narcotics can be given in pill form or by skin patches. Sometimes disease of other organs may be confusing the endometriosis picture, so a multidisciplinary approach may be necessary. In such a situation, urologists may diagnose and treat interstitial cystitis, physical therapists may treat abdominal and pelvic muscle syndromes, and psychologists may evaluate and treat the mental well-being of the patient and her family. The main risk associated with treatment as pain management centers is the development of tolerance to narcotics and eventual narcotic addiction in some patients. Some patients attending pain management centers also worry that the cause of their pain is not being treated.

For women who are unwilling to do nothing, and who have exhausted reasonable efforts at medical therapy, surgical treatment of endometriosis is the only choice. This is not to say that all women with endometriosis should receive medical therapy before they undergo surgical treatment, however. Medical therapy given before a surgical diagnosis often delays the correct diagnosis of pelvic pain, which usually requires surgery to determine. Medical therapy also treats only symptoms; it does not eradicate the underlying disease. If a doctor provides a patient with a thorough discussion as part of the informed consent process before beginning treatment, many women might reject any effort at medical therapy as only a "Band-aid" approach compared to the results with surgical therapy.

Pain management centers

Clinics in which several types of practitioners try to control the symptoms of endometriosis (and other pain-causing diseases) by using a multidisciplinary approach.

48. Do advanced stages of endometriosis respond to medical therapy?

The answer to this question depends what is meant by "response." If it is taken to mean that disease is eradicated, then no stage of endometriosis responds to medical therapy. If it is taken to mean that symptoms respond temporarily during treatment, then earlier, less severe stages of endometriosis have some chance of responding. Studies show that symptoms associated with advanced stages of endometriosis respond poorly to medical therapy, including treatment with hormone-bearing IUDs. Advanced cases of endometriosis require surgical treatment.

PART FOUR

Surgical Treatment

Does hysterectomy cure endometriosis?

How is intestinal endometriosis treated?

Why do women with endometriosis seem to have so many surgeries?

More . . .

49. Does hysterectomy cure endometriosis?

No. Endometriosis is found most commonly in sites that are separate from the uterus, so removal of the uterus will not have any effect on endometriosis elsewhere. Removal of the uterus—a procedure called **hysterectomy**—is sometimes necessary for treatment of uterine problems that don't respond to simpler treatment. Uterine problems that can be resolved by this surgical procedure include heavy or irregular bleeding, painful uterine cramps, uterine pain due to adenomyosis, symptomatic fibroid tumors, and cancer. If symptoms originating in the uterus are mistakenly attributed to endometriosis, removal of the uterus might seem to be good "treatment" for endometriosis because those uterine symptoms will be gone, although the endometriosis symptoms may persist. This is why it is necessary to separate pain caused by endometriosis from pain caused by the uterus or some other organ.

If a gynecologist believes that endometriosis is caused by reflux menstruation, then it would be a small leap of faith to imagine that removal of the uterus might be important in eliminating future formation of endometriosis. Because endometriosis is not really caused by reflux menstruation, however, this hope is misplaced. There is no scientific proof that removal of the uterus is important in preventing future endometriosis. Endometriosis can certainly exist and continue to cause symptoms after removal of the uterus.

50. What is ablation, and how is it related to Sampson's theory of origin of endometriosis by reflux menstruation?

Ablation is removal of diseased or unwanted tissue by surgery or other means. In regard to surgical treatments for endometriosis, it is a generic term that could conceivably

Hysterectomy
Surgical removal of the uterus.

Endometriosis involving the uterus is uncommon. Removal of the uterus only will usually leave behind 99% of the disease.

Ablation
Removal of diseased or unwanted tissue by surgery or other means.

include thermal destruction techniques such as laser vaporization, electrocoagulation, harmonic scalpel, endocoagulation, or argon beam coagulation. While the term can also be used to mean "cutting a disease out of the body," when "ablation" is used in reference to the surgical treatment of endometriosis it implies thermal ablation techniques only.

All thermal ablation techniques have similar actions on cells. Using heat generated by light (laser), heat generated by resistance to electron flow (electrocoagulation and argon beam coagulation), heat generated by sonic vibrations (harmonic scalpel), or heat from a hot surgical probe (endocoagulation), water and protein inside cells are targeted. The cell can literally explode because of the rapid boiling of the water inside it if the power of the instrument is high, or it may slowly coagulate like an egg white if instrument power is set to a low level.

While ablation techniques have some potential for destroying endometriosis, the depth of burn they produce can be quite shallow, often less than 2 mm. When used in a rapid fashion, the depth of burn may only be the thickness of a human hair or two. Considering that many lesions of endometriosis extend deeper than 2 mm into the tissue, it is no wonder that undertreatment with ablation techniques is common. The efficacy of ablation techniques has not been validated by reoperating on treated patients to see whether endometriosis has been eradicated or reduced in amount. Ablation techniques violate common surgical sense and remain unproven.

Medicine, like spoken language, is practiced best when done in a precise fashion. Thus the term "ablation," when it is used to describe so many different surgical techniques, is representative of the imprecision of thought and action that have led to the confusion that is

If a doctor misdiagnoses uterine symptoms as endometriosis symptoms, then when hysterectomy cures the uterine symptoms, the doctor may think that hysterectomy is good treatment for endometriosis.

Surgical ablation of endometriosis could include laser vaporization, electrocoagulation, endocoagulation, harmonic scalpel coagulation, or argon beam coagulation.

SURGICAL TREATMENT

Ablation of endometriosis does not allow the doctor to know how deeply en- dometriosis invades tissue.

the unfortunate hallmark of some modern treatments of endometriosis. Unrelated techniques are lumped together under one label, which implies to doctors and patients alike that all of these techniques are equivalent—which is not necessarily so. In this case, imprecise language is a proxy for imprecise surgery. "Ablation" defines no precise technique or endpoint of surgery:

- The depth of penetration of endometriosis remains unknown because the surgeon makes no attempt to explore the lesion by dissection.

Ablation of endometriosis cannot be used safely over the ureter, bowel, or large blood vessels.

- The required depth of destruction there- fore remains in question, so undertreatment is common, although the surgeon can claim that complete treatment has occurred.

- The surgeon must guard against burning too deeply in certain areas lest underlying vital struc- tures be damaged, again inviting undertreatment.

- Because no pathology report is obtained, the sur- geon can claim that any particular disease has been destroyed.

The effective- ness of abla- tion has not been studied by repeat laparoscopy to see how well it works.

- After incomplete treatment of endometriosis, the surgeon can blame recurrent or persistent pain on Sampson's theory of reflux menstruation rather than on incomplete surgical treatment.

The relationship between the incomplete surgical treat- ment resulting from thermal ablation techniques and Sampson's theory of origin of endometriosis is a sinister symbiosis. Sampson's theory of origin of endometriosis predicts that all surgical treatments will fail, and abla- tion techniques provide that failure.

51. What is excision of endometriosis?

Excision is a surgical term that means "to cut out." Excision of various diseases has been practiced by surgeons for centuries. It makes good common sense to remove a disease from the body rather than leaving it in. Excision of endometriosis means that the abnormal tissue is cut out of the body. Before the introduction of birth control pills or GnRH agonists, laser vaporization, electrocoagulation, or any of the other modern therapies that now exist, a surgeon had only one option to offer a woman with endometriosis who wanted to maintain her fertility: the surgeon could open the abdomen with laparotomy and cut the disease out of the body. Excision is, therefore, the oldest treatment for endometriosis.

Excision at laparotomy is done with scissors and electrosurgery. Excision by laparoscopy can be performed with scissors, electrosurgery, carbon dioxide laser, or fiber laser. With carbon dioxide laser, the laser beam is delivered through the carbon dioxide distending the abdomen. With fiber laser, the laser energy is delivered down a fiber-optic bundle.

Excision gives the surgeon the best opportunity to go around and underneath all disease, ensuring more complete removal of the abnormal tissue. Because some endometriosis may extend several centimeters beneath the visible surface, this surgical technique is ideal for treating endometriosis. Excision can be used anywhere in the body endometriosis occurs. Most cases of excision of endometriosis, including most cases of intestinal endometriosis, can be performed laparoscopically.

Excision

A type of surgery in which diseased parts are cut out of the body.

SURGICAL TREATMENT

Excision is the only treatment for endometriosis that allows complete removal of either superficial or deep disease anywhere in the body.

52. Is excision of endometriosis easy to do?

Excision of extensive cases of endometriosis is more difficult than cancer surgery.

Excision of endometriosis can be simple to do when only the peritoneum is involved. This thin, transparent, flexible covering of the abdominal and pelvic cavities can be readily pulled away from underlying structures and the endometriosis cut away rapidly.

The ability to pull the tissue away from underlying structures to protect them is one of the advantages of excision over thermal ablation techniques. Most often, surgeons using thermal ablation techniques do not pull the peritoneum away from the underlying vital structures, but rather just burn the peritoneum where it is in place over these structures. This increases the likelihood of unintentional burns to these underlying structures, so surgeons using thermal ablation techniques have the impossible task of judging exactly how deeply to burn to destroy all disease while not burning so deeply as to damage underlying structures. These concerns are greatly reduced with excision.

When endometriosis is associated with scar tissue around it, the peritoneum can be thicker and sometimes fused to the underlying structures such as the ureter. In these cases, the surgeon must carefully pry the endometriosis away from underlying structures. This is done mechanically with small metal instruments. After the thickened, fibrotic peritoneum is freed from surrounding structures, it can be excised.

53. How are endometrioma cysts of the ovary removed?

Cyst

A cavity filled with fluid. The fluid is not necessarily watery.

Endometrioma **cysts (Figure 7)** can range in diameter from about 1 cm to 20 cm or larger. They are frequently stuck to the bottom of the pelvis, uterus, and intestines by scar tissue that forms in response to the irritation of the cyst.

To remove an endometrioma cyst, the ovary with the cyst in it is freed from surrounding scar tissue, and the cyst is punctured and drained of its fluid. The wall of the cyst is then pulled out from the ovary, leaving normal ovarian tissue behind. To prevent the ovary from sticking back down to the pelvis over the ureter, the ovary can be suspended from the pelvic sidewall with absorbable sutures.

If an endometrioma cyst is just punctured and drained, there is almost a 100% chance that the cyst will simply reaccumulate fluid. Even if the surgeon tries to burn the interior of the cyst wall in an effort to destroy it, the failure rate is more than 90% with this technique.

The ovary is not the most common site of pelvic involvement. However, if the ovary is involved by endometriosis, there is an almost 100% chance that the patient has disease elsewhere in the pelvis. Thus, if only ovarian endometriosis is treated, there usually has been undertreatment of the patient's disease. Compared to women who have endometriosis but no ovarian disease, women with endometrioma cysts of the ovary tend to have more extensive disease elsewhere in the pelvis, as well as an increased chance of intestinal involvement.

Ovarian endometriosis is a marker for more extensive pelvic and intestinal endometriosis. Women with ovarian endometriosis almost always have disease elsewhere in the pelvis.

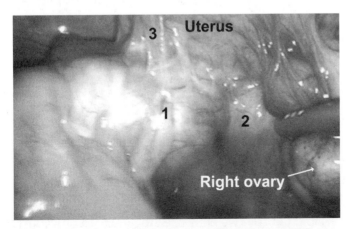

Figure 7 The left ovary involved by an endometrioma cyst (1), obliteration of the cul-de-sac (2), and massive adhesions (3)

54. How is intestinal endometriosis treated?

The large bowel has four layers. The outer layer (the serosa) is basically an extension of the peritoneum. There are two muscle layers, an outer longitudinal and inner circular. Finally, the inner lining of the bowel is called the **mucosa**. Endometriosis of the bowel always starts on the serosa and extends to varying degrees into the muscle layers, resulting in spherical scarring and retraction and formation of new smooth muscle around the endometriosis. The mucosa is almost never involved by endometriosis.

The wall of the small bowel is thinner and contains three functional layers: the serosa on the outside, a thin muscle layer, and the mucosa on the inside. The diameter of the small bowel is less than that of the large bowel, as the name implies. As a consequence, the small bowel is more susceptible to partial obstruction due to scarring and retraction due to endometriosis.

Bowel resection is used for treatment of intestinal endometriosis. The word **resection** means to remove a part of something. If endometriosis is very superficial on the outer bowel wall, it can be removed by superficial bowel resection, much like removing a mole from the skin. If the outer muscle layer of the bowel is involved by endometriosis, a partial-thickness bowel resection is used. If the outer and inner layers of bowel muscle are involved, the dissection may go all the way to the inside of the bowel, in which case a full-thickness bowel resection is occurs. When large tumors of endometriosis are present, or when multiple nodules occur side by side, then it may be necessary to remove a segment of bowel and put the two ends back together—a procedure

Mucosa

A layer of tissue that has the ability to produce a secretion that can resemble mucus.

Cyclic rectal bleeding with menses is rare in women with intestinal endometriosis, but when present it suggests that the endometriosis has invaded the entire thickness of the bowel wall.

Bowel resection

TThe surgical removal of a portion of bowel.

Resection

To remove a piece of tissue surgically. Synonymous with excision.

called a segmental bowel resection. Most patients with intestinal endometriosis do not need a segmental bowel resection, however, and most cases of intestinal endometriosis can be treated laparoscopically.

Patients with a suspicion of intestinal endometriosis may receive a **bowel prep** before surgery and antibiotics during and for a short time after surgery. It is not necessary to perform a colostomy for treatment of intestinal endometriosis, although a temporary colostomy may be necessary in rare cases when postoperative complications arise due to leakage of bowel contents through suture or staple lines.

Bowel prep
A fluid that is more concentrated than normal intestinal contents and is used to prepare a person for bowel surgery.

55. How is endometriosis of the diaphragm treated surgically?

Symptomatic endometriosis of the diaphragm is always located far on the rear side of the diaphragm, and it always penetrates the full thickness of the diaphragm. The full extent of diaphragmatic endometriosis cannot always be seen using a laparoscope placed in the umbilicus, because it's often hidden by the liver. For this reason, a second, smaller laparoscope may be placed under the margin of the right ribs so that the surgeon can see the entire rear side of the diaphragm.

A colostomy is not needed to treat intestinal endometriosis.

Occasionally, the surgeon may see small, superficial "sentinel" lesions when the laparoscope is placed in the umbilicus. Although these lesions can potentially be destroyed by thermal ablation techniques, they do not cause the main symptoms of endometriosis, so any pain relief will be incomplete. Medical therapy for diaphragmatic endometriosis is ineffective.

More than 90% of diaphragmatic endometriosis affects the right diaphragm.

Symptomatic diaphragmatic endometriosis has always invaded the full thickness through the diaphragm.

Because symptomatic diaphragmatic endometriosis is always full thickness, it is necessary to remove a full-thickness piece of diaphragm to ensure removal of all endometriotic tissue. The problem is that performing laparoscopic surgery in this area is virtually impossible because it is so hard to reach with the scope. Inserting a thoracoscope into the right chest allows the surgeon to see the areas where endometriosis has invaded the full thickness of the diaphragm, and it becomes possible to pick up the area of involvement and remove it by stapling across the normal diaphragm adjacent to the lesion, then cutting the lesion off. The problem with this technique is that there may be more lesions of endometriosis on the abdominal side of the diaphragm that won't be seen; if they are left in place, they may potentially cause symptoms later. Given that endometriosis of the diaphragm seems always to start on the abdominal side of the diaphragm, it makes more sense to approach it from the abdominal side so that the entire extent of the disease can be seen.

Posterior

An anatomical term. As a person is viewed standing, posterior is toward the back side of the body.

Because laparoscopic surgery on the **posterior** or rear side of the diaphragm is virtually impossible, obtaining the best results requires that a laparotomy incision be made running along the lower margin of the ribcage. The surgeon can then put his or her hand into the upper abdomen and retract the liver downward, allowing the endometriosis to be seen. This tissue can be cut out with scissors and the hole in the diaphragm closed with suture. A small suction drain may be left in for a day or two.

Treating sentinel lesions will not help symptoms very much.

Although the recovery from this type of laparotomy is longer than the recovery after laparoscopy, the payoff for the patient is it achieves nearly 100% pain relief. After resection of the diaphragm, breathing is normal (or improved, because many patients have difficulty breathing with their disease in place) and patients can participate in normal athletic activities without shortness of breath.

Women with symptomatic diaphragmatic endometriosis always have extensive pelvic disease and usually have extensive intestinal disease as well. Treatment of these patients requires major surgery to be performed on several organ systems.

Kim's story:

I had right chest and shoulder pain since the age of 24. Each month, it would begin just before my flow and get incredibly bad during my flow. I could barely take a breath, it was so painful. As years went by, the pain began to occur earlier and earlier each month, until I was hurting sometimes 2 weeks before my flow and the week of the flow itself. So I had only 1 week where I felt "normal," which was just a little bit of pain.

I had every test they could think of, including an EKG for heart attack, but everything was "normal." [The doctors] thought it might be endometriosis because it was so tied to my menstrual flow, but the drugs they tried didn't work. I finally had a laparoscopy. They saw some endometriosis and lasered it, but that didn't seem to do anything for my pain. I was going crazy and felt like I was doing something wrong, and that it was my fault that I wasn't getting better.

I finally had a big surgery where they cut under my ribs and removed the part of the diaphragm that was involved. The difference was like night and day. I could tell in the recovery room waking up from surgery that the pain was gone. It was a miracle. I wish I'd done this years ago. I can do whatever I want without having to think about chest pain. I don't have to take any hormones or anything.

The symptoms of diaphragmatic endometriosis are so well recognized that testing is not needed to be certain of the diagnosis.

56. *How is endometriosis of the bladder treated?*

Endometriosis of the bladder is easy to see and frequently easy to treat.

The bladder has three layers: the serosa, which is the peritoneum covering the bladder; the muscularis, or muscle layer; and the mucosa, or inner layer. Endometriosis of the bladder might not cause any symptoms if it consists of a superficial deposit on the peritoneum over the bladder. This type of disease is very easy to remove because the peritoneum carrying the endometriosis can be picked up and trimmed off.

Antibiotics during surgery are unnecessary for treating bladder endometriosis. Urine is sterile, so even a full-thickness resection carries a low risk of infection.

When endometriosis invades the bladder muscle, it may cause bladder cramping when the bladder is full or when it is emptying. Because symptomatic bladder endometriosis rarely penetrates all the way through to the mucosa, urological examination with a cystoscope or bladder x-rays is usually normal. Endometriosis involving the bladder muscle always starts from the outside of the bladder, so the disease can be readily seen by the laparoscopic surgeon. When it invades the muscle, a hard, spherical nodule is present, but it may not always be obvious unless the bladder is palpated.

Although superficial endometriosis could theoretically be treated with thermal ablation techniques, deeper endometriosis will require removal of a part of the bladder wall—a procedure called a partial cystectomy. While it has the same name as the surgical procedure to remove an ovarian cyst, the surgery on the bladder is obviously a totally different procedure. First, the surgeon cuts into the normal soft bladder muscle around the tougher nodule. The nodule may be removed by taking out only the involved muscle fibers, but some nodules are large enough that they reach almost to the mucosa. The dissection in such a case will go all the way through the bladder wall, and the part of the bladder wall carrying the nodule will be removed. The bladder is sewn closed, and a urinary catheter is used for several days to keep the bladder empty so the hole in the bladder wall has a chance to heal and become watertight. Bladder function is normal after healing. This partial cystectomy surgery can be done laparoscopically fairly easily.

57. How is endometriosis of the ureter treated?

The ureter is the muscular tube that carries urine from the kidney to the bladder. Most people have one kidney on the left side and one kidney on the right side of the body. Women with endometriosis have a slightly higher rate of a urinary tract abnormality called **renal agenesis**, in which a kidney fails to form on one side and the ureter on that side is absent as well. Because one kidney is enough for normal human survival, this condition doesn't cause any problem, although that person cannot be a kidney donor! Sometimes a kidney is drained by two ureters, one draining the top of the kidney and the other draining the bottom. When this situation is present, the ureters usually join together low in the pelvis before entering the bladder. Thus a woman with endometriosis may have zero, one, or two ureters on either side.

When the ureter is involved by endometriosis, it is always related to a nodule of endometriosis in the uterosacral ligament on the same side. Typically, the uterosacral ligament is less than an inch from the ureter. When a nodule of endometriosis develops in this ligament, it enlarges, causing the distance between the uterosacral ligament and ureter to decrease. Scar tissue can extend outward from the nodule, surrounding the ureter and

Renal agenesis

A urinary tract abnormality in which the kidney and ureter are missing on one side of the body.

Endometriosis invading the ureter is quite rare.

67

trapping it. When this happens, the scar tissue may constrict slowly over time and interfere with the ureter's ability to empty urine into the bladder.

When the nodule in the uterosacral ligament is larger, it may grow directly into the side of the ureter facing the center of the body. The endometriosis invades the muscle of the ureter and can begin to constrict the diameter of the ureter by this invasion. If the ureter doesn't drain urine out of the bladder properly, the build-up of back-pressure in the kidney may eventually kill the kidney function permanently on that side. Constriction of the ureter can occur so slowly that the kidney dies a silent death, only to be discovered after the fact.

When scar tissue surrounds the ureter, surgery involves cutting the scar tissue off of the ureter and then removing the nodule of the uterosacral ligament that caused the problem in the first place. When endometriosis invades the muscular wall of the ureter, the segment of ureter that is involved is removed, and the ends of the ureter are sutured back together over a **stent** (a hollow plastic tube that ensures drainage of urine past the suture line into the bladder). The length of ureter removed is usually less than 1 cm. When a stent is used, it is removed several weeks later in the urologist's office. All of these surgeries can be done laparoscopically by an experienced surgeon.

Stent

(In ureteral surgery) A hollow plastic tube that ensures drainage of urine past the suture line into the bladder.

58. Do I need a hysterectomy as part of my treatment for endometriosis?

Not usually. Removal of the uterus is sometimes necessary for treatment of uterine symptoms such as cramps or other uterine pain, heavy or irregular bleeding, or cancer. By contrast, removal of the uterus has no important role to play in treatment of endometriosis because in most women, the uterus is not involved by endometriosis. Also, the uterus has no role in the development of endometriosis, so hysterectomy as a means to "prevent" endometriosis is not warranted.

59. Do I need my ovaries removed as part of my treatment for endometriosis?

The ovaries are not the most common site of involvement by endometriosis, so most women will not require surgery to be performed on the ovaries. If superficial endometriosis on the ovaries is present, it can be evaporated with electrodessication, one of the only useful techniques possible with electrocoagulation. If an ovarian endometrioma cyst is present, it can usually be removed without having to remove the ovary. The ovaries are the most difficult pelvic area to cure of endometriosis with one surgery because small endometrioma cysts may be present but hidden somewhere in the ovary.

Removal of the ovaries is not necessary to treat pelvic or intestinal endometriosis.

There are certain situations in which removal of the ovary makes sense. Women with very large cysts and women with several endometrioma cysts may have only a paper-thin shell of tissue left after removal of such cysts. This tissue is so thin that sutures can tear through it and the ovary can't be reconstituted into a reasonable volume, or the thin shell may be prone to bleeding that cannot be controlled easily. In such cases, it would be best to remove the remainder of what was once called an ovary.

In addition, women who have multiple surgeries to treat recurrent cysts in the same ovary may do better if that ovary is removed, as long as the other ovary seems reasonably healthy. Repeated surgeries on the ovaries to remove cysts may rarely result in premature menopause in some women. This likelihood is related to age, meaning that it is more likely to occur in older women. Nevertheless, premature menopause as a result of repeated removal of ovarian cysts can occur in women in their late twenties as well.

Nancy's story:

I guess I was born too soon. In my day, doctors didn't think twice about telling a patient what was going to be done. Options were few and far between. When I was 29, I had a total abdominal hysterectomy and removal of the ovaries. That took care of my uterine cramps, but I had a sneaking suspicion that I still had endometriosis because of some persistent pain. Sure enough, almost 20 years later I had laparoscopic surgery and removal of endometriosis that had been left in so long before. Well, I guess better late than never.

60. Why do women with endometriosis seem to have so many surgeries?

Inadequate surgical treatment of symptomatic endometriosis often necessitates at least one more surgery to remove all of the endometriotic tissue.

There are several reasons for the frequency of surgery. Many surgeries involve thermal ablation techniques that don't burn deeply enough to destroy all disease, virtually guaranteeing persistent symptoms. Some surgeries are performed to just look at the endometriosis but do nothing else—an approach that guarantees symptoms will persist. Some surgeries are done to remove something else that is not involved by endometriosis, such as the uterus, fallopian tubes, or ovaries. Women can still have symptomatic disease after removal of all the pelvic organs, however—even if they are not taking estrogen replacement therapy. Some surgeries are performed to look at endometriosis after medical therapy is completed. Because there is no medicine that eradicates endometriosis, the results of this surgery are almost pre-ordained: Endometriosis will still be present.

Juliet's story:

I can't believe I had my fourth laparoscopy for this cruddy disease and I still have pain. After my second surgery, I went to see a doctor who is well known for cutting out the disease. He was a [jerk], so I saw his associate, who seemed confident and nice. She did my surgery and removed lots of endometriosis, but I knew by one week after surgery that I was still having the same old endometriosis pain.

I was a good girl and waited until I was all healed so they couldn't tell me [my pain] was related to healing. Then I went to the doctor who had burned my endometriosis out with my first two surgeries, and he said I probably had endometriosis back again, and if I wanted to have children that I should have another surgery. So I did. And guess what? There was endometriosis everywhere! The lining of the pelvis had grown back shorter than before and it had endometriosis all over it. He used a laser to burn it all out and said it was all gone at the end of surgery.

Long story short, by two weeks after surgery, I was having the same pain that I'd had all along. None of the surgeries for endometriosis had changed my pain. I contacted another "expert" in endometriosis in another state who doubted any more surgery for endometriosis could help and that the problem was probably with my uterus all along. But I know my body, and I know what endometriosis pain feels like. I'm worried that I have occult endometriosis that just hasn't been found. I want to have kids and I know I don't want a hysterectomy.

Juliet's words carry the probable answer to her pain: None of the treatments for endometriosis has ever helped her pain, which makes it very likely that endometriosis may never have been the cause of a lot of her pain, as suggested by the latest surgeon she consulted.

Janet's story:

I was told that I had the most resistant case of endometriosis in the world. I'd had 15 surgeries and I was still in pain. I'd had laparoscopy for diagnosis, laparoscopy with laser burning followed by medical treatment, laparoscopy with electrical burning followed by more medical treatment, laparoscopy to see if the disease was still there (it was), laparoscopy with laser again followed by three medicines at the same time, and so on. Nothing worked. I was told that endometriosis is incurable, and that the reason I was hurting is because it always comes back. Then I went to a doctor who cuts the disease out. He removed all of the areas that looked abnormal and none of them showed endometriosis on the pathology report! He must have missed some, though, because I still hurt. Maybe I have occult endometriosis.

Rigorous biopsy of suspected lesions at each surgery would dispel much of the confusion around endometriosis.

Or maybe Janet never had endometriosis in the first place! If all women had aggressive laparoscopic excision of their disease, the number of repeat surgeries would be markedly reduced. Not only would the best surgical treatment be done the first time, but pathology reports at follow-up surgeries could help precisely define whether endometriosis was present. That information would help many patients get off the endometriosis merry-go-round and allow them to pursue other causes of their pain. Janet's story shows in a strange way that endometriosis truly can be "incurable": A doctor can give it to you simply by diagnosing this condition even when you don't have it. Biopsy proof of the presence or absence of disease is crucial to proper care. Without it, both doctors and patients will remain confused, and some patients may continue to believe they have endometriosis even when it has been proven that they don't.

61. Which serious complications are possible with surgical treatment of endometriosis?

The complications that may arise with endometriosis surgery are the same no matter where in the body surgery is done. The main risks are bleeding, infection, damage to other organs, formation of scar tissue, and reoperation to fix a complication. There are also risks associated with the use of anesthesia during the surgery, including pneumonia.

The risks of endometriosis surgery are the same no matter where in the body the surgery is done.

Bleeding is obvious at surgery when it is occurring. It may be controlled surgically by any number of means, including coagulation, ligation with suture, or application of a metal clip. One of the problems with blood vessels is that the muscles in their walls can be in spasm at the end of surgery. This spasm can stop bleeding from some vessels even if the end of the vessel is open. As a consequence, the surgical field can look bloodless at the conclusion of surgery, only to have a vessel in spasm relax later, allowing bleeding to occur within a few minutes or a few hours after completion of surgery.

The risk of significant complications is less than 4% when the patient is in experienced hands.

Bleeding can sometimes occur 2 or 3 weeks after surgery, although this problem is uncommon. Normal wound healing takes 6 to 8 weeks to be completed. Before healing has been completed, blood vessels that have been coagulated, sutured, or clipped may not have formed all of the dense scar tissue that will keep the vessel closed forever. As sutures dissolve, as coagulated areas soften, or as clips shift, the incompletely healed vessel may open through the still-weak cut end and bleeding may occur. If the vessel is large enough, reoperation may be necessary. Although most postoperative bleeds do not require reoperation, patients require careful observation, preferably in the hospital, to see which direction things will turn.

Infection occurs when bacteria begin to grow in the surgical site. This bacterial invasion may occur either in the skin or deeper down inside the body. Although an antiseptic prep is applied before any cut is made during surgery, it is impossible to sterilize the skin or the vagina, so bacteria can enter the body from those surfaces.

The body is able to fight off a certain number of bacteria. This ability to defend against bacteria varies on the basis of the strength of the person's immune system as well as on the basis of the virulence of the bacteria.

Bacteria like to grow in blood. In the laboratory, for example, bacteria are often grown on sheep's blood in agar dishes. Given this propensity to flourish in blood, the combination of even a small postoperative bleed and some bacteria may set the stage for an infection to occur.

Infections are uncommon after laparoscopic surgery for endometriosis because the scope is usually not inserted into the vagina in such procedures. Infections are more common if the uterus is removed, because the vagina is opened and some bacteria may still be present there that can gain entrance up inside the pelvis.

Some patients may benefit from the administration of prophylactic antibiotics to prevent infections, including individuals who are obese. Because overuse of antibiotics can induce the emergence of resistant bacteria, there is little reason to give these medications prophylactically to all patients, especially given that most surgical patients will not develop an infection. The risk of infection can also be reduced without resorting to antibiotics. During surgery, lots of irrigation fluid can be used to rinse the pelvis of any bloody fluid that might provide bacteria with a growth medium. Inserting a drain after surgery can help remove any bloody fluid that might remain, as well as help remove any infection that might try to produce pus. Also, the drain can be used to take bacterial cultures from the pelvis after surgery if an infection is suspected.

Damage to some organs may be intentional, such as when endometriosis is removed from those organs, or it may be unintentional. Unintentional injuries to adjacent structures may not be completely avoidable. Endometriosis and the scar tissue it can produce can be so intimately connected to a vital structure that damage to the structure is inevitable, even if the surgeon anticipates the danger and proceeds extremely cautiously. Fortunately, if the injury is recognized and repaired at once, there is typically no long-term problem.

Sometimes a partial injury occurs to an organ or structure, which then breaks down several days after the surgery. Such an event may necessitate reoperation. A partial-thickness injury would typically not be as obvious as a full-thickness injury, which would generally invite early discovery and repair. Even so, rare occurrences of a full-thickness injury to the bowel, bladder, or ureter going unidentified and unrepaired at surgery have been reported. Such injuries lead to almost immediate postoperative pain and usually require early repeat surgery to identify and fix the problem.

Eileen's story:

I realize that complications are a possible risk of surgery, and I signed a consent form before surgery to acknowledge this. I didn't expect it to happen to me, though, or to take so long to find and fix.

I had a severe case of endometriosis with involvement of my bowel and tissue around my ureters. The bowel endometriosis was removed and my ureters were cleaned off. By 24 hours after surgery, I was sick as a dog. They took me back to surgery expecting to find a leak in my bowel, but they didn't find it. The bowel was fine. There was some cloudy fluid in my pelvis and they thought I'd developed an infection, so they took cultures, left a drain in, and started me on different antibiotics. This didn't help my problem, though.

I was in severe abdominal pain for 2 days and had difficulty breathing. They kept giving me pain medicine, but it wasn't doing any good: The drain kept putting out fluid. Finally, my doctor injected a dye in my bladder to see if it would come out the drain. The drainage tube kept putting out the same color fluid. He then injected a dye in my IV line that would turn my urine blue as it came out of the kidneys. When the drainage coming out of my abdomen turned blue, they knew that a ureter had been damaged.

I was taken back for a minor surgery, and they found a small leak in both ureters! They put tubes up my ureters and almost immediately my pain was better. I was in the hospital for 3 weeks with all of this going on.

PART FIVE

Other Causes of Pelvic Pain

What is adenomyosis?

What is interstitial cystitis?

What is irritable bowel syndrome?

More . . .

62. Is all pelvic pain due to endometriosis?

It would be too simple if all pelvic pain were caused by endometriosis. Sometimes doctors are too quick to assume that endometriosis is the cause of a patient's pain if she has been diagnosed with endometriosis in the past.

There are several well-defined causes of pelvic pain other than endometriosis. When you consider that the pelvis contains not just the female reproductive organs but also the bladder, bowel, muscles, and bones, it is not surprising that each of these organ systems might be associated with some type of pain that can occur all by itself or with other conditions, including with endometriosis. This section of the book provides a brief overview of some of the other causes of pelvic pain and explains how they are diagnosed and treated. Further information should be obtained from your doctor or from your own research.

The gynecological organs, for example, can be associated with pelvic pain. The uterus can hurt because of adenomyosis or fibroids. Even a uterus that is entirely "normal" can hurt, causing uterine cramping with the menstrual flow. The ovaries can form cysts that can hurt, although some cysts cause no pain. Cysts can cause pain by rupturing, bleeding, growing, or undergoing ovarian torsion.

Ovarian torsion

A condition in which an ovary twists around its blood supply.

In **ovarian torsion**, an ovary twists around its blood supply. Mild enlargement of the ovary, typically by a cyst, is necessary before ovarian torsion will occur.

An analogy would be to consider a balloon. When a balloon is empty, it has little mass. If you hold the open end of the balloon and try to twirl the closed end, not much will happen because the closed end doesn't have much mass or moment of inertia. But now fill the balloon with a cup of water, hold it by the open end, and twirl the end with water in it. The balloon will twirl around several times with enough force.

In the same fashion, a normal ovary doesn't have enough mass to twist on its "stalk," but an ovary with a moderate-size cyst might have enough mass to twist as time goes by. Twisting can occur with normal body movements and posture changes, or it may occur as a result of intestinal peristalsis gently pushing the ovary around.

Ovarian torsion is most common with cysts between 3 and 6 cm in diameter. Larger cysts tend to become wedged in position in the pelvis, so there's not enough room for them to twist. The treatment for ovarian torsion is to untwist the ovary, drain and remove the cyst, and then suspend the ovary from the side of the pelvis with sutures so it isn't quite so mobile. Often an ovary that looks "dead" during surgery will look fine after being untwisted. Rarely the ovary may be strangled so long by torsion that it dies and needs to be removed.

63. What is adenomyosis?

Adenomyosis (**Figure 8**) is a benign disease of the uterus. This distant relative of endometriosis is one of the leading causes of non-endometriotic pelvic pain. In adenomyosis, the endometrium, which lines the interior cavity of the uterus, invades the muscular wall of the uterus. This invasion can be superficial just beneath the endometrium, or it can pass completely through the muscle wall and erupt on the outside surface of the uterus.

Adenomyosis can be diffuse, like termites in a wall, or it can exist in clumps or nodules called adenomyomas. **Adeno-** is a medical prefix referring to glands; "myoma" is a medical term referring to muscle. Under the microscope, adenomyosis can be seen to consist of glands resembling the lining of the uterus surrounded by muscle fibers.

Pain due to endometriosis typically starts in early teenage years. Pain due to adenomyosis typically starts in a woman's late twenties to early thirties.

Adenomyosis

A benign disease in which the endometrium, which lines the interior cavity of the uterus, invades the muscular wall of the uterus.

Adeno-

A medical prefix that means relating to glandular tissue.

Because of their microscopic similarities and similar symptoms, adenomyosis and endometriosis have somewhat of a shared history. In the early twentieth century, researchers were just beginning to describe what we would today call deeply invasive endometriosis. They were already aware of adenomyosis in the uterus. Because deeply invasive endometriosis was composed of glands and stroma surrounded by muscle tissue, these severe forms of endometriosis were called **adenomyomas**. Thus adenomyomas of the rectovaginal septum, adenomyomas of the umbilicus, adenomyomas of the inguinal canal, and adenomyomas of the bladder were all so named because of this characteristic microscopic appearance. (The correct Latin plural for adenomyoma is *adenomyomata*, as you recall from your childhood classical education.) For its part, adenomyosis of the uterus resembled endometriosis in the sense that glands of the endometrium were misplaced into the uterine muscle. Thus, in the past, adenomyosis has been called *endometriosis interna*, meaning that it is internalized in the uterus, as opposed to *endometriosis externa*, which refers to endometriosis that is scattered around the pelvis.

Adenomyoma

The first name given to deeply invasive endometriosis.

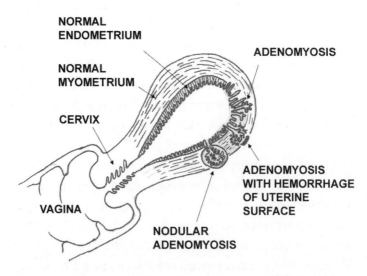

Figure 8 Adenomyosis of the uterus. Most cases remain hidden in the wall of the uterus.

64. How is adenomyosis diagnosed?

The patient's history provides key information when diagnosing adenomyosis. Whereas endometriosis can begin to cause pain in the early teenage years, adenomyosis begins to cause pain in a woman's late twenties. Because adenomyosis is a uterine condition, it is associated with uterine symptoms. Therefore, uterine cramps before or during the menstrual flow are common. These may be mild or severe, and they sometimes begin a week or two before the flow starts. Some women may have cramps all month long at a reduced level, with extreme menstrual aggravation of cramps possible. Irregular or heavy uterine bleeding can also occur with adenomyosis.

The physical exam can provide some evidence for or against adenomyosis. The uterus can be normal size with adenomyosis, or it may be slightly enlarged when there is extensive uterine involvement. The chief helpful finding during pelvic exam, however, is uterine tenderness that reproduces some or all of the patient's symptoms. A nontender uterus does not rule out adenomyosis, because sometimes adenomyosis may be present without symptoms, or the exam might have been on a "good day" when symptoms were absent. If palpation of the cul-de-sac results in tenderness that reproduces the patient's pain, and in such a patient if the uterus is nontender, then endometriosis may be the more likely culprit.

Imaging studies such as ultrasound, CT, or MRI are often performed to evaluate pelvic pain. If adenomyosis is superficial and has not invaded very far into the uterine muscle, it will not show up on any scan. If the disease is more extensive, the uterus may be enlarged symmetrically and the muscle may seem mottled on the scan. The rear muscular wall of the uterus is the area most commonly involved by adenomyosis, perhaps because it is in the embryologic pathway of organogenesis of the pelvic organs. If the rear wall of the uterus appears thicker than the rest of the uterus, it represents slightly stronger evidence that adenomyosis is present. Occasionally, adenomyosis can be nodular and can look like a fibroid tumor on the scan.

Scans have only two possible results: normal or abnormal. A normal scan does not exclude disease; an abnormal scan doesn't mean that the cause of the disease has been isolated or indicate what the disease is if it has been isolated. With either a normal or abnormal scan, the patient will still be hurting and will have to make a decision about treatment based primarily on the severity of symptoms and whether she wants to try to conceive in the future.

65. How is adenomyosis treated?

Adenomyosis is usually diagnosed with certainty only after hysterectomy, which is the only treatment that is always successful.

Removal of the uterus is the only treatment that is 100% effective in eliminating the symptoms of adenomyosis. The disease typically is diffuse throughout the uterus, so there is no way to remove just the adenomyosis. Occasionally, a single nodule of adenomyosis is present that could potentially be removed, much like trimming out a fibroid tumor of the uterus. However, diffuse adenomyosis may still be present and be left behind.

There is no medical treatment that eradicates adenomyosis. Because the disease is so difficult to diagnose without hysterectomy, patients might receive treatment with birth control pills or ovarian suppressive agents like those used to treat endometriosis. The response to medicines is temporary, however. Even if symptoms are reduced during treatment, they inevitably return after treatment stops.

In women with recurrent pain after previous surgical excision of endometriosis, adenomyosis is frequently the culprit.

66. What is primary dysmenorrhea?

Dysmenorrhea refers to abnormal and difficult menstrual flows. This somewhat broad term doesn't necessarily refer to uterine cramps with the flow, but can also include pain during the flow from non-uterine causes including endometriosis. Dysmenorrhea can occur *secondary* to uterine diseases such as adenomyosis or fibroids, or *secondary* to diseases outside the uterus such as endometriosis or interstitial cystitis. With *primary* dysmenorrhea, no other cause seems to exist, and the problem is generally with the uterus itself. In such a condition, a uterus that otherwise is entirely normal can be the cause of severe cramps and pain. Even if the uterus is removed in an attempt to eliminate the symptoms, the diagnosis comes back "normal" from the pathology examination. Thus even a "normal" uterus can cause severe pain, possibly because something biochemically or hormonally abnormal is happening at the level of the cell that we're not smart enough to know about.

67. What are uterine fibroids?

Uterine fibroids are smooth muscle tumors that can develop from the wall of the uterus. These tumors usually have a spherical shape. If they hang on a stalk off the outer surface of the uterus, they are called **pedunculated**. If they grow within the muscular wall of the uterus, they are called **intramural**. If they grow next to the endometrium, they are called **submucosal**.

Dysmenorrhea
Abnormal or difficult menstrual flows.

Uterine fibroid
A smooth muscle tumor that develops in the wall of the uterus; known more formally as a leiomyoma uteri.

Pedunculated fibroid
A fibroid that hangs by a stalk from the outer surface of the uterus.

Intramural fibroid
A fibroid whose main volume arises from the middle of the muscular uterine wall.

Submucosal fibroid
A fibroid that is next to the mucosa, the inner lining of the uterus.

Fibroids are rarely malignant. These tumors can be as small as a grain of sand or very large and weigh many pounds. A woman may have a single fibroid or several dozen fibroids. The medical term for fibroids is *leiomyomata uteri*, which is Latin for "smooth muscle tumors of the uterus."

68. What are the symptoms of uterine fibroids?

Uterine fibroids may cause pain and bleeding. Ultimately, the symptoms experienced depend on the sizes of the fibroids and their locations in the uterus. Fibroids smaller than 2 cm in diameter may cause no symptoms.

When fibroids grow within the muscle layer of the uterus, they can irritate the uterine muscle and produce uterine cramping. These cramps may just accompany the menstrual flow or they may occur all month long, but with aggravation during the flow.

When fibroids grow near the endometrial lining of the uterus, they can cause irregular or heavy bleeding. Pedunculated fibroids don't seem to cause much in the way of symptoms unless they are very large. Large fibroids may cause a sense of pelvic pressure or fullness. They may press on the bowel or bladder and affect urination and bowel movements. In some women, these tumors press on nerves passing through the pelvis and cause pain in the distribution of that nerve.

Fibroids may not prevent conception, but larger tumors may interfere with growth of the fetus or interfere with delivery by altering the position of the baby in the uterus. Fibroids can grow in response to estrogen, but some fibroids cease growth after reaching a certain size. Fibroids generally cause symptoms beginning when a woman is in her late twenties and may continue until she reaches her early fifties (that is, when she reaches menopause).

69. How are uterine fibroids diagnosed?

Fibroids can sometimes be felt on pelvic exam as irregular protrusions from the surface of the uterus, which is normally smooth like a small pear. Fibroids larger than 1 cm show up well on ultrasound, CT, or MRI scans. Ultrasound is the type of scan that is most commonly done for the diagnosis of fibroids. Not all "fibroids" on scans turn out to be fibroids, however. Nodular adenomyosis may look like a fibroid on a scan, and the difference may become apparent only when surgery is performed to remove the "fibroid."

70. How are uterine fibroids treated?

No medicine is available that can make fibroids go away permanently, although the low estrogen state caused by treatment with GnRH agonists may reduce their size somewhat. The high costs and significant side effects of GnRH agonists make long-term treatment with these drugs impractical. After menopause, the ovaries no longer produce significant estrogen, and fibroids may shrink to a virtually undetectable size. The average age at which women experience menopause is approximately 50, but most women with fibroids are not interested in waiting years or decades for menopause to resolve the problem.

Fibroids can often be felt on pelvic exam in the office as lumps and bumps of various sizes that distort the normal smooth shape of the uterus.

Because no medicine eradicates fibroids, something surgical must be done to them. There are three main choices: (1) remove the fibroid, (2) remove the uterus, or (3) choke off the blood supply to the fibroid.

Myomectomy

Surgical removal of a fibroid from the uterus.

Palpation of the uterus at laparotomy can find more fibroids than ultrasound can.

Removal of a fibroid surgically is called a **myomectomy**. This procedure can be done laparoscopically, but a better choice is frequently to open the abdomen by laparotomy. The reason for this preference is that fibroids can be very small and hidden within the uterus. By opening the abdomen, the surgeon can palpate the uterus with his or her fingers and find tiny fibroids that did not show up on any scan. It is not unusual for ultrasound to reveal several larger fibroids and then for the surgeon's fingers to find many more. Whether these smaller fibroids would ever grow and cause symptoms cannot be predicted, but many women would want the most complete job done if they are going to the trouble, expense, and risk of having surgery for fibroids. The risk of developing a new symptomatic fibroid in the future is less than 25%.

Another advantage of removing fibroids by laparotomy is that the procedure can be done more quickly and the resulting defect in the uterus repaired more quickly than with laparoscopy. This issue is important both for reducing blood loss and for ensuring a better repair of the uterus. The blood supply to fibroids varies, and the location of the feeder vessels cannot be predicted. Thus, when a fibroid is removed, bleeding can come from anywhere around the edge of the fibroid. Injecting medicine to help constrict blood vessels or placing a tourniquet around the uterus to restrict its blood supply temporarily can help reduce blood loss, but nothing works better than quickly clamping off bleeders and suturing them. To help conserve blood even more, a device called a Cell Saver can be used during surgery. Blood that is suctioned out of the pelvis during surgery can be collected, piped to this machine for cleaning, and then transfused back into the patient after the end of surgery. These actions reduce the need for transfusion with banked blood. If the hole that is created in the uterus to remove fibroids is deep, some obstetricians may recommend delivery by cesarean section in the future to reduce the risk of uterine rupture during labor.

For women who have completed their childbearing career, removal of the uterus is probably the best treatment for symptomatic uterine fibroids. This surgery can often be done laparoscopically and leads to less blood loss because the blood supply to the uterus is in predictable anatomical locations. These blood vessels can be closed by suture or electrocoagulation before they are cut, so a hysterectomy may be almost bloodless. Once the uterus has been separated from its pelvic attachments, the fibroids can be removed from it by operating vaginally. When the size of the uterus has been reduced in this way, it can then be removed vaginally. The recovery after laparoscopic surgery is less painful and about 4 weeks shorter than after a laparotomy.

Some fibroids may be treated by choking off the blood supply to the uterus—a process known as **uterine artery embolization (UAE).** In this case, an interventional radiologist inserts a long catheter into one of the arteries in the legs and threads the catheter into the arteries supplying the uterus. Metal particles or other blocking agents can be injected through the catheter; these substances enter the arteries and block them, thereby depriving the fibroids of much of their blood supply.

In UAE, the radiologist will try to get the catheter as close as possible to the larger fibroids so that the blood supply just to the fibroid is interrupted, but sometimes some of the normal uterine tissue can be affected. Rare cases have been reported of loss of the uterus due to massive obstruction of it blood supply.

Removal of the uterus is simpler and associated with less blood loss than removal of fibroids.

Uterine artery embolization (UAE)

A procedure that shrinks the size of uterine fibroids by blocking the arteries to the fibroids, thereby depriving them of much of their blood supply.

Although this technique can be successful for targeting the larger fibroids that can be seen on scans, smaller fibroids will go largely untreated. Thus the question remains about whether they will cause problems in the future. Successful pregnancies have been reported after UAE, but many radiologists would recommend that this procedure be done only in women who have completed their childbearing career because of uncertainty about the ability of the uterine wall to withstand growth during pregnancy or to tolerate labor and delivery.

71. What is interstitial cystitis?

Interstitial cystitis (IC) is an inflammatory condition of the urinary bladder. It is far more common in women than men, and approximately 25% of patients with this condition are younger than 30 years of age.

Although many patients are familiar with the term "cystitis," referring to bladder infections caused by bacteria, IC is not caused by an infection. Instead, it results form irritation of the bladder muscle by direct contact with urine. The inner lining of the bladder, called the mucosa, protects the underlying muscle from urine collecting in the bladder. With IC, this protective layer develops holes in it that allow the urine to make more direct contact with the bladder muscle, which then becomes irritated by the minerals and other chemicals found in the urine.

72. What are the symptoms of interstitial cystitis?

When the bladder muscle is irritated by IC, the bladder can hurt and the bladder muscle can spasm, leading to the feeling of having to empty the bladder even when

Interstitial cystitis (IC)

An inflammatory condition of the urinary bladder that is caused by irritation of the bladder muscle by direct contact with urine.

Interstitial cystitis seems to be more common in women with endometriosis and can confound the diagnosis of endometriosis.

it's not full (urgency) or the need to empty the bladder too often (frequency). These are some of the same symptoms that can be produced by bacterial infections of the bladder. Symptoms may be aggravated during the menstrual flow or by certain foods in the diet. Women with endometriosis may have a higher risk of also having IC.

73. How is interstitial cystitis diagnosed?

Suspicion for IC develops when a patient has symptoms of serial urinary tract infections (UTIs), which are treated with antibiotics unsuccessfully. The urine culture is negative for bacterial growth, however, and it eventually becomes clear to the doctor and patient that this is not a true UTI. On pelvic examination, the only characteristic finding is tenderness in the region of the bladder.

An office procedure is sometimes performed to diagnose IC. A catheter is placed into the bladder and an irritative fluid, such as potassium iodide, is injected into the bladder. If this reproduces the symptoms that the patient experiences at home, it is taken as evidence of IC.

Another way of diagnosing IC is called **bladder hydrodistention**. In this procedure, a cystoscope (an optical tube that resembles a laparoscope) is inserted into the bladder, and fluid is pumped into the bladder until it is distended to three or four times its normal maximal capacity. This procedure is done under a general anesthetic because it would be so uncomfortable otherwise. The bladder is allowed to remain in this overdistended state for several minutes, and then the fluid is drained while the doctor looks at the bladder wall with the cystoscope.

With hydro-distention, the bladder is distended by liquid to 3 or 4 times its normal volume to look for changes associated with IC.

Bladder hydrodistention

A procedure for diagnosing interstitial cystitis in which an optical tube is inserted in the bladder, fluid is pumped into the bladder, the fluid is drained, and the physician then examines the bladder wall.

Trabeculation

A strand of bladder muscle that has become thicker than normal; a sign of interstitial cystitis.

Glomerulation

A tiny area of capillary bleeding; a sign of interstitial cystitis.

Signs of IC include **trabeculations**, strands of thick bladder muscle that have become bigger than normal because of the bladder "exercising" itself by squeezing too frequently and too forcefully. The doctor also looks for **glomerulations**, tiny areas of capillary bleeding. As the bladder empties, the blood from these fragile capillaries can begin to fill the bladder, mixing with the clear irrigation fluid like a red snowstorm. The degree of IC is judged by how irritated the bladder appears to be on the basis of this bleeding. A normal bladder will have few trabeculations and almost no glomerulations or bleeding.

Other possible causes of bladder symptoms need to be considered, including bladder stones, bladder cancer, UTIs, STDs, or endometriosis.

74. How is interstitial cystitis treated?

Because the cause of IC is not known, a cure for this condition is elusive and treatments target symptoms rather than seeking to eradicate the disease. The same hydrodistention technique used to diagnose IC may provide some temporary reduction in symptoms. Given that the cause of IC is incompletely understood, long-term treatment is necessary. This treatment is directed at two goals: (1) relief of symptoms and (2) regrowth of the protective inner lining of the bladder.

Many approaches to treatment of IC are used because no one thing works for every case. Altering the diet to eliminate foods that trigger symptoms can be helpful. Experimentation is necessary to determine which foods an individual must avoid, although caffeine, acidic foods, and salt are frequently culprits. Sometimes birth control pills will reduce symptoms, although their effectiveness varies.

Bladder retraining is sometimes helpful. It requires that the woman try to hold her urine in her bladder for at least 15 minutes after the onset of urgency. Visiting the doctor's office frequently to have bladder instillations with medicines may also be helpful. These medicines may include sodium bicarbonate, DMSO, local anesthetics, heparin, and pentosan polysulfate (Elmiron®). Some patients may wish to do their own bladder instillations at home.

Oral medicines include Elmiron®, which is the only FDA-approved medicine for treating IC and works to help the lining of the bladder to regrow. Neuromodulators may alter how pain is processed by the nerves, and sedatives may help relax the patient. Some oral medicines that are used in UTIs act like a local anesthetic in the urine, and these may be helpful for relieving IC symptoms as well. Using a cystoscope, Botox® can be injected into the bladder muscle in several points, which may temporarily reduce the irritability of bladder action. IC is increasingly being diagnosed and other treatments are being actively studied.

Botox can be injected into the bladder wall during cystoscopy to help reduce bladder muscle irritability.

75. What is irritable bowel syndrome?

Irritable bowel syndrome (IBS) has a precise diagnosis and a loose diagnosis. The precise diagnosis is the Rome criteria requiring at least 12 weeks a year when a patient has abdominal pain or discomfort that has at least two of the following three features:

- Pain is relieved by bowel movements.

- Onset of symptoms is associated with a change in frequency of bowel movements.

- Onset of symptoms is associated with a change in form or appearance of bowel movements.

Irritable bowel syndrome (IBS)

A condition characterized by intestinal cramping, bloating, change in stool, nausea, diarrhea, and constipation. IBS may be caused by a disease such as endometriosis irritating the outside of the bowel, or it may have no identifiable cause.

Abdominal and pelvic inflammation caused by endometriosis can cause symptoms of IBS, which may clear up after surgical removal of endometriosis.

The loose definition of IBS is probably more commonly used and refers to a loose amalgam of intestinal symptoms such as bloating, intestinal cramping, abdominal pain, nausea, vomiting, diarrhea sometimes alternating with constipation, or excess gas. Endometriosis of the pelvic surfaces or of the intestinal tract can irritate the abdominal cavity and the intestines, so these "looser" symptoms of IBS are common in women with endometriosis.

IBS typically does not cause blood in the stool, fever, weight loss, or pain that awakens people from sleep.

76. How is irritable bowel syndrome diagnosed?

IBS is typically a diagnosis of exclusion: Other diseases are ruled out until no other obvious explanation for symptoms exists. The most important diseases to rule out are Crohn's disease of the small intestine, ulcerative colitis, and intestinal cancer. Abdominal scans, barium enemas or swallows, and colonoscopy are the most common tests to diagnose bowel problems; combinations of these tests may be performed as necessary. Virtual colonoscopy, which is a variant of high-definition three-dimensional CT scanning, is increasingly being used. Also growing in popularity is a small camera the size of a pill that is swallowed and that takes pictures as it passes through the intestinal tract.

77. How is irritable bowel syndrome treated?

Because the cause of IBS is not known, there is no precise treatment for it. Instead, therapy is directed at trying to manage symptoms. This most commonly involves altering the diet to eliminate foods that trigger symptoms. Reducing stress may help, as may increasing the amount of fiber in the diet. Anticholinergic drugs that calm the intestines down may also be helpful. Over-the-counter medicines to control diarrhea may be occasionally helpful.

78. What are adhesions?

Adhesions are a form of scar tissue. Whenever there is sufficient injury or inflammation in the body, the body eventually heals by laying down scar tissue. While the terms "adhesions" and "scar tissue" are somewhat synonymous, a slight distinction could be made based on appearance. Scar tissue consists of a flat scar, such as a scar on the skin from surgery or a burn. Adhesions, by contrast, are bands of scar tissue that stick things together (thus the name).

Adhesions most commonly occur somewhere inside the body, but they can also be seen on the skin, such as burn contractures around joints where thick bands of adhesions may extend from one side of the joint to the other, pulling the joint closed. Inside the body, adhesions can range in visual appearance from transparent curtains between structures (**Figure 9**) to thick areas that look like someone threw strong glue into the body and things became stuck to it in a big wad.

> **Adhesions**
> A form of scar tissue that "glues" two or more surfaces together.

> *Scar tissue is the body's normal response to injury.*

79. How are adhesions related to endometriosis?

Adhesions form in response to inflammation or injury. Certain cases of endometriosis can be especially inflammatory so adhesions can form as a response. Ovarian

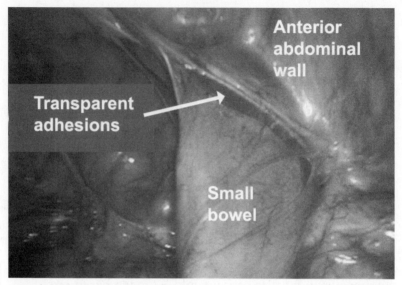

Figure 9 A transparent curtain of adhesions binding a portion of small bowel to the anterior abdominal wall. This type of adhesion is easily treated.

endometriomas are especially prone to forming adhesions. This type of adhesion is usually a confluent type that glues an entire side of the ovary to the pelvic sidewall like two pieces of paper glued together. Obliteration of the cul-de-sac occurs when the rectum sticks forward to the rear of the cervix due to adhesions, with invasive endometriosis under virtually all the surfaces. Adhesions can tighten up over time, so adhesions that were once fairly loose and caused no symptoms can become tighter and cause symptoms later.

80. Do adhesions cause pain?

Adhesions can cause pain, although they do not necessarily always do so. When two or more surfaces become stuck together by adhesions, the connection can put traction on the things that are stuck together, causing pain.

With endometriosis, adhesions may cause pain when an ovary becomes stuck to the side of the pelvis because of the irritation caused by an ovarian endometrioma cyst. If the cyst grows in size, it can pull on the adhesions the way inflating a basketball under a blanket can pull around the edges of the blanket. A cyst by itself may not hurt, and adhesions by themselves don't always hurt, but the two together in the same area can increase the chance for pain.

Some patients who have pain due to adhesions describe an increase of the pain with certain movements or postures, such as reaching overhead, which stretches the adhesions. Sometimes adhesions can affect the surface of the intestines, gluing intestines down when they are supposed to be free to glide around like a bowl of cooked spaghetti. If a loop of intestine is stuck down in the wrong way by even one well-placed adhesion, the bowel may become kinked so that intestinal contents may not be able to get through, leading to symptoms of partial or complete bowel obstruction. The small bowel is much more likely to develop such an obstruction than is the large intestine.

Adhesions binding surfaces together can tighten over time, sometimes causing symptoms months or years after they form.

81. Do adhesions cause infertility?

If the ends of the fallopian tubes are scarred shut by adhesions so the egg can't be picked up, then adhesions can definitely cause infertility. When adhesions are present in the pelvis, they do not necessarily keep the egg from being picked up by the end of the fallopian tube. The pelvis is somewhat like a salmon spawning bed: an egg pops out of an ovary and falls into the small amount of free fluid normally present, which can allow it to be swept past the end of either fallopian tube for pickup. The egg is tiny and the fluid can carry it between curtains of adhesions so that conception has a chance to occur.

Thus the real question is not necessarily whether adhesions are present. They are ugly to look at but may not affect fertility and are rather biologically inert. The real question is whether the inflammatory process that left the adhesions is still active. An active inflammatory disease such as endometriosis is more likely to affect fertility than adhesions left by a process that is no longer active.

82. How are adhesions diagnosed?

At surgery, adhesions may look like anything from transparent plastic wrap, to wet tissue paper, to wads of glue. The thinner manifestations of adhesions do not show up on any scan. If bowel obstruction is present, a simple abdominal x-ray may show loops of small bowel dilated by gas and snaking down to a point, beyond which the bowel gas pattern is normal. The kink in the bowel keeps the gas from going through as easily as it should, and the transition point on the x-ray between dilated bowel and normal bowel is the precise location of the adhesion, although the adhesion itself doesn't show up. Thicker masses of adhesions may show up on ultrasound or CT scan as ill-defined masses.

Surgery is the most accurate way to diagnose adhesions and see what type of problems they are causing.

83. How are adhesions treated?

Because no medicines treat adhesions, surgery is required for treatment, a process called **adhesiolysis**.

Adhesiolysis

The surgical treatment of adhesions. "Lysis" means to break apart or cut.

Two types of adhesions are distinguished: (1) two or more surfaces may be joined by flexible adhesions that hang like ropes, cobwebs, or threads; or (2) two or more surfaces may be glued together like sheets of paper. The first type of adhesion can be treated by cutting across each end, like cutting both sides of a rope hanging between two points. The adhesion can then be removed from the body. There is only a small chance of this type of adhesion recurring because the surgery to remove it isn't very traumatic to the body.

The second type of adhesion is more problematic. The surfaces must be pried or cut apart. This fairly traumatic procedure leaves raw surfaces all over the place, which can invite re-formation of the adhesions in the same places.

One thing the surgeon must keep in mind is why the adhesion formed in the first place. Adhesions that form after surgery are a different problem than adhesions that form because of underlying biologically active endometriosis.

84. Can adhesions be prevented?

Sometimes. When there are raw areas left by prying two surfaces apart during adhesiolysis, it is necessary to separate those two surfaces during healing; otherwise, they will very likely stick together again. For example, if an ovary is stuck to the side of the pelvis due to the inflammation of an endometrioma cyst within it, after surgical treatment the ovary can be suspended from the adjacent round ligament so that the raw area on the sidewall won't come in contact with the raw area on the ovary. This will prevent the ovary from becoming strongly adherent to the sidewall in most cases.

New adhesions are more likely to form following laparotomy than laparoscopy.

When the cul-de-sac is obliterated by the effects of underlying invasive and biologically active endometriosis, the rectum is stuck by adhesions to the back of the cervix. If the rectum is separated from the back of the cervix and nothing is done about the underlying endometriosis, there is a chance the adhesions will just re-form because the endometriosis is still present and active. To reduce the chance of adhesions re-forming, all endometriosis should be removed so that the only adhesions that will try to form are the inert type that occurs after surgery.

Various commercial agents have come on the market that claim to prevent adhesions. One of these has been found to produce adhesions in laboratory animals, and another has been taken off the market because of severe reactions leading to more adhesions and bowel obstruction. Others remain on the market, but some surgeons are hesitant to use them because of variable and small margins of success and problems with previous agents. Some surgeons recommend leaving extra irrigation fluid in the pelvis at the end of surgery, with the idea that the fluid will tend to float things around so that they might be less likely to stick together.

Early second-look lap-aroscopy has been found to decrease the ultimate amount of adhesions.

Early second-look laparoscopy is sometimes used in patients who have a history of repeated operations for adhesions. The efficacy of second-look laparoscopy is based on the fact that adhesions may re-form within 7 to 14 days after they are lysed. Early second-look lap-aroscopy is done about 7 days after lysis of adhesions. At this time, the adhesions are just forming and are soft compared to what they might be like 6 months later. These soft adhesions can be broken apart without much effort, with less surgical trauma. Repeat operations on patients having second-look laparoscopy for adhesiolysis show that this approach is effective.

Some patients may have a loop of bowel that repeatedly sticks down after adhesiolysis. As the number of surgeries on that area of bowel increases, the area of bowel becomes increasingly more abraded and, therefore, is more likely than ever to stick to something again. It may be necessary to remove the segment of bowel that has been repeatedly re-injured so that only clean, smooth bowel remains behind. This type of bowel would be much less likely to stick down again.

85. Can musculoskeletal problems cause pelvic pain?

Pelvic muscles can go into spasm and cause pain just like a "Charlie horse" in the calf. This spasm may often be an involuntary reaction to pelvic pain from some other cause. Pelvic floor muscle dysfunction can be diagnosed by palpating the main pelvic muscles during pelvic examination. The muscles on one side may seem tighter and more tender than the muscles on the other side. Treatment can involve treating other causes of pain that might have contributed to the spasm in the first place. Also, physical therapy and internal massage may be helpful, while injection of Botox® into the spasming muscle may have benefits as well.

PART SIX

Fertility Issues

Can endometriosis cause infertility?

Does pregnancy cause endometriosis?

Does pregnancy cure endometriosis?

More . . .

Randomized controlled trial (RCT)

The "gold standard" of medical proof of the relative efficacy of one treatment over another, or over using nothing at all (placebo). Patients with a disease and who are similar to one another in most other respects (such as age, height, weight, duration of illness, and severity of disease) are assigned to one treatment group or another by randomization. The patients undergo treatment and are followed for a certain length of time to see if there is any difference in the results of the treatments studied.

Selection bias

A situation in which the way a group is selected for study influences any conclusions reached from that study. Selection bias has contributed to the confusion surrounding endometriosis.

86. Can endometriosis cause infertility?

Yes. This has been shown by a **randomized controlled trial (RCT)** showing that surgical treatment of infertility improved the conception rate over doing nothing at all. Some women with untreated endometriosis can get pregnant, however. Generally, though, women with endometriosis take longer to conceive than women without endometriosis. This means they have fewer children in their lifetime.

87. Does pregnancy cause endometriosis?

This sounds like a stupid question, but it's not. Many articles published in medical journals about endometriosis describe studies in which most of the women have already conceived and delivered babies. If you were to look at this fact alone, you would naturally wonder whether endometriosis was caused by pregnancy because "so many fertile women get it." This conclusion would be challenged, though, by those who would say that this conclusion was reached in error because of selection bias. **Selection bias** means that the way a group is selected for study influences any conclusions reached from that study.

A nonmedical example of selection bias would be counting vehicles passing on a road. If the count were done between 8:00 A.M. and 9:00 A.M. when children are being delivered to school, it might seem that most cars on the road are minivans driven by women. But if the count was done in the evening, the cars would seem to be of all types and their drivers of both sexes. Thus the time of day when the count takes place could introduce selection bias that affects the outcome. It might be more accurate to count all cars passing for 24 hours, although that result could vary depending on the day of the week, because schools are usually closed on weekends. So it might be better to do the counting for an entire 7-day week, unless it's during Christmas break when school is out. In that case, it might be better to do the counting for an entire month, unless it happens to be during summer when school is out and semi-trailers are allowed on the road. Counting every vehicle passing over an entire year, day in and day out, 24 hours a day, would be the best way to get an idea of what type of cars use the road, since this is the only time period that would remove all selection bias. This would also give a large number of cars that would solidify the results, because a small number might not necessarily be representative of what happens on the road.

How does selection bias affect what we know about endometriosis? First, early studies on endometriosis were very small, usually involving fewer than 30 patients, and these studies focused on the most severe manifestations of the disease (which were the most obvious and most readily discovered) in patients who were typically in their mid-thirties. One notable study focused mostly on women who did not have endometriosis. Fertility declines with age, so if we add up all these little factoids, we deduce the following: Looking at a small number of women in their mid-thirties with the most severe form of endometriosis (although some did not have endometriosis, but we'll include them anyway) would produce the inevitable observation that these women seemed to have lower fertility. That was the observation made in those groups of women at that time.

Seeing these results, the study authors concluded that endometriosis caused fertility and then went on to make another unsupported corollary conclusion that pregnancy protects against endometriosis. This statement is the inverse of the statement that pregnancy causes endometriosis. Yet no one questions that pregnancy protects against endometriosis because it has been accepted without question or true scientific proof for many decades.

On the face of it, both statements are ridiculous because they are based on separate populations of patients who were somehow selected for study. For example, you can be sure that women with endometriosis entering an office with a sign over the door reading "Infertility treated here" will tend to look infertile compared to women in pain who visit a general obstetrician-gynecologist in a rural town who then get diagnosed with endometriosis. Which is the "correct" population that is more representative of women with the disease? Some might say the women in the rural town. If most of those rural women with endometriosis had been pregnant, then the conclusion could be reached that pregnancy causes endometriosis.

Depending on how you select a group for study, almost anything can be thought to be true.

Another effect of selection bias is that early thought on endometriosis frequently focused on infertile patients, leading to the notion that infertility was the most common symptom of the disease. We now know that pain is the most common and most specific symptom of endometriosis.

88. Does pregnancy cure endometriosis?

No. There is no evidence whatsoever for this statement, even though this "leap of faith" conclusion has been passed along for many decades. It reaches back to the notion that women who have been pregnant seem to have a lower chance of having endometriosis than women who have not been pregnant. While an association may exist between endometriosis and not being pregnant, this does not mean that a cause-and-effect relationship is present. Even so, a cause-and-effect relationship has been accepted over the years by virtue of sheer rote repetition, aided and abetted by the observation that endometriosis pain may be reduced during pregnancy.

89. Does medical therapy of endometriosis improve fertility?

No. Medical therapy seems to decrease fertility because by the time a woman completes 6 months of medical therapy and resumes ovulating a month or two after that, she will still have all her endometriosis but will be about 9 months older and, therefore, less fertile due to the age-related decline in fertility that affects all women. There is no medicine approved by the FDA for treating infertility in women with endometriosis. Surgery is the only treatment for infertility due to endometriosis. Women can attempt conception beginning 5 weeks after surgery.

90. Does surgery for endometriosis improve fertility?

Yes. This outcome has been shown by a randomized controlled trial, which is considered the gold standard of scientific proof. In one study, one group of infertile women with endometriosis got surgery directed against their disease, while the other group received "sham" surgery where laparoscopy was performed but nothing was done to the endometriosis that was found. The surgically treated group had twice the conception rate of the untreated group. A second similar study, however, found no improvement in fertility following surgery.

Fertility declines with age in both women and men. A woman is most fertile between ages 15 and 25. A delay of 6 months or more in conception attempts due to medical treatment of endometriosis results in a greater reduction of fertility than the 5-week delay following surgery for endometriosis.

FERTILITY ISSUES

Nevertheless, women with endometriosis who are infertile and who seem to have no other treatable cause of infertility should consider surgery as soon as possible. Surgery does not reduce fertility.

The longer a woman has tried unsuccessfully to conceive before surgical treatment of her endometriosis, the lower are her chances of conception following surgery. There are two reasons for this. First, endometriosis may not have been what was keeping the woman from becoming pregnant. Remember that women can conceive even if their endometriosis is untreated. Thus, the longer a woman with endometriosis goes without conception, the less likely it was the endometriosis that was keeping her from getting pregnant and the more likely that some other cause of infertility was operating silently in the background. Surgery for endometriosis will not affect this silent cause of infertility, which may never be discovered in a particular woman. Second, the longer a woman has tried to conceive before surgery, the older she will be at the time of surgery. Because fertility declines with age, these older women are less fertile simply for that reason.

The beneficial effects of surgical treatment of endometriosis last for years.

Many doctors mistakenly believe that there is a "window" of 6 to 9 months following surgery during which a woman must conceive; otherwise, the beneficial effect of surgery is lost. This notion derives from observation of graphs of the conception rate after surgery, which rises for the first 9 months or so and then levels off. This is a classic misinterpretation of data, however (**Figure 10**). Such a graph actually includes two populations of patients. In one group, endometriosis is the only thing keeping them from conceiving. When their disease is removed, members of this group conceive in the first several months after surgery, producing the rapid rise in the conception

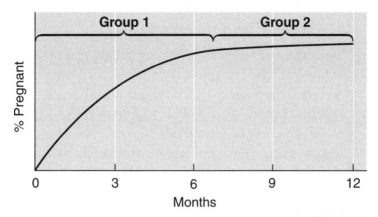

Figure 10 The fertility curve after surgery for endometriosis is the result of operating on two populations of patients: those whose infertility was caused only by endometriosis (group 1) and those women with endometriosis whose infertility was caused by something else (group 2).

rate seen in the "window." The second group of infertile patients has endometriosis but it is not preventing conception; rather, some other cause of infertility is present, whether known or not. Surgery will remove these patients' endometriosis but not treat the real cause of their infertility. Members of this group will still have difficulty getting pregnant at any time after surgery and, therefore, contribute to the flatter part of the conception rate graph seen beyond 9 months.

The benefits of surgery on infertility are long-lasting. This effect is seen best in women who had excision of endometriosis as teenagers. Most were unmarried and not trying to conceive at that time in their lives. Years later, long after the 9-month "window" has closed, after marrying and starting families, these women have an almost normal conception rate curve.

The longer a woman has been infertile before surgical treatment of endometriosis, the less likely she is to conceive after surgery.

91. Why do doctors say that pregnancy is good for endometriosis?

Just because something is repeated by doctors doesn't make it correct. Doctors aren't immune from herd mentality.

This statement is what doctors are taught and what they read—but that repetition does not necessarily make it correct. Like many myths, if something is repeated often enough by enough people, it begins to be accepted as truth. Those who oppose rote repetition of dogma and who demand facts are sometimes looked down upon. After all, how could the entire group belief be wrong?

Gina's story:

I was in pain and I wanted to get pregnant. I had been trying for 5 years. I was diagnosed with severe endometriosis at laparoscopy and was told that I should get pregnant since that was good treatment for endometriosis. Hello! I had been trying to get pregnant, including taking medicine to make me ovulate better.

I was given injections for 6 months after surgery that reduced my pain a lot, but the pain started coming back within a few weeks of stopping it. I was back at square one, except we had less money because insurance didn't pay the $500 per month that the medicine cost. Finally, I had laparoscopic excision of endometriosis. I had given up on getting pregnant; I just wanted pain relief. I could tell as soon as I woke up in recovery that the pain was gone! It was a miracle. What was even more miraculous is that I conceived 4 months after surgery without taking medicines and now I have a beautiful baby girl. Why don't doctors get it?

92. Is a fertility doctor the best type of doctor for treating endometriosis?

Not necessarily. The best choice of physician to treat a condition depends on what the condition being treated is. With respect to treating symptoms of pain, any doctor can prescribe medical therapy for endometriosis, so you don't have to be an expert in endometriosis or infertility to treat the symptoms with medicine. This is one of the marketing points of drug manufacturers. Unfortunately, when the treatment stops, the pain comes back in most women because the disease is still present.

Infertility specialists are called **reproductive endocrinologists**. One of the main things they have to offer infertile women with endometriosis is **assisted reproductive technology (ART)** techniques such as in vitro fertilization (IVF), augmentation of ovulation, intrauterine insemination (IUI), or **intracytoplasmic sperm injection (ICSI)**. These procedures can bypass some of the deleterious effects of endometriosis and get many women pregnant, although the endometriosis may continue to cause painful symptoms in the future.

There is some evidence that the results of ART may improve if endometriosis has been surgically treated. Not all infertility specialists do a lot of surgery. In fact, there was a time when reproductive endocrinologists actively avoided doing surgery because they were afraid that a woman's infertility problem would be worsened after surgery because of postoperative scar tissue formation that could keep her from conceiving. (Think about that for a minute and you will see the false logic in that concern.) As a result, very few reproductive endocrinologists would consider themselves expert in treating endometriosis surgically. Because surgery is so important in

FERTILITY ISSUES

Reproductive endocrinologist

A doctor who subspecializes in treatment to assist women in getting pregnant. After completing standard specialty training in obstetrics/gynecology, a physician completes an additional 2-year fellowship to become a reproductive endocrinologist.

Assisted reproductive technology (ART)

Any technique that is used to enhance the chance of conception, such as in vitro fertilization (IVF) or intrauterine insemination (IUI).

Intracytoplasmic sperm injection (ICSI)

A technique that forces fertilization of the egg by injecting sperm directly into the egg.

In-vitro fertilization can help some women with endometriosis conceive without surgery, although these patients may still be bothered by endometriosis pain after delivery.

Excision of endometriosis may improve IVF results and also treats endometriosis pain.

treating either pain or infertility due to endometriosis, a fertility specialist may not be the best type of doctor to treat a woman with endometriosis.

Surgery for endometriosis can be the most difficult surgery in the human body because endometriosis can invade most vital organs of the pelvis and abdominal cavity, up to and including the diaphragm. Endometriosis surgery is far more difficult than cancer surgery. The best type of doctor to treat endometriosis is a surgeon or a team of surgeons who can treat the disease wherever it occurs.

PART SEVEN

Heredity

Is endometriosis hereditary?

Is there a gene for endometriosis?

Will my daughter get endometriosis
if I have it?

More . . .

93. Is endometriosis hereditary?

It is likely that several or many genes are responsible for the cause of endometriosis.

To a certain degree, endometriosis is certainly hereditary. In some families, endometriosis can be found in three generations of women. First-degree relatives of women with endometriosis also have an increased chance of having the disease. But does this increased risk arise simply because the women in the family have become familiar with endometriosis and its symptoms and are quick to seek out medical advice when they experience similar symptoms, or does it reflect a true genetic basis for the basis?

Because endometriosis is a very common disease, one need not look very far into a family tree to find several women with the disease. Yet, in other families, only one woman is known to have the disease. Just from superficial observations like this, we might suspect that endometriosis potentially is hereditary, but it might also arise sporadically apart from a hereditary influence. But if it is a disease that might arise sporadically very commonly, then endometriosis might seem to be hereditary when it's not. And then there is the question of whether we really know exactly whether every woman in a family tree does or does not have endometriosis because it's impossible to do the surgery necessary to diagnose endometriosis in 100% of women.

As this discussion suggests, using family trees to try to plot the hereditary nature of endometriosis is of limited clinical value. To really know about **heredity** and endometriosis, we would need to know more about the genome of women with endometriosis.

Heredity

The process by which genetic traits are passed from parents to their offspring.

94. Is there a gene for endometriosis?

Several genes most likely affect the development of endometriosis. If you learned about genes in school, you may have a fairly basic idea that they impart characteristics to offspring. A very simple model of gene activity is the notion of the autosomal dominant gene. In this model, if one parent has a particular autosomal dominant gene, it will be passed on to 50% of the offspring, and any offspring receiving that gene will display whatever characteristic the gene codes for. In autosomal recessive inheritance, both parents carry a particular gene that has the potential to cause a disease. The parents don't display the disease because the disease is expressed only if the person carries a matched pair of these genes. Offspring have a 25% chance of receiving the particular gene from both parents, thereby receiving a matched pair and displaying the disease.

These simple models of gene function are somewhat like an on/off light switch. In reality, genetics turns out to be more complicated in many cases. Genes can be turned completely on, turned partially on, or turned off. The function of genes can be altered by the action of one or several other genes, each of which could be influenced by the actions of other genes, and so on. Therefore, gene expression can be more like a dimmer switch on a light with an infinite number of levels of interaction possible.

Genetic studies are being done on women with endometriosis and their families, and it seems clear that the actions of several or many genes are important in the origin of the disease. This is an emerging field that currently has no useful clinical application; certainly, there is no **gene therapy** currently available for endometriosis. Given the complexity of the emerging picture, gene

Genes can be off, on, or partially on. Genes can affect the function of other genes. Nongenetic material in DNA can affect gene function.

Gene therapy of endometriosis would make far more sense than any current treatments, but it is probably many years away.

Gene therapy

Replacing defective genes with normal genes to correct a disease state; or inserting a new gene that corrects the actions of a defective gene.

therapy for this disease remains years or decades away. Gene therapy would give a more sensible way of treating the disease than the fruitless attempts of modern therapy to use hormonal influence. Stay tuned to this station.

95. Will my daughter get endometriosis it if I have it?

She may or may not. Because endometriosis seems able to sporadically strike almost anyone, the more important question is whether your daughter is having pelvic pain, with or away from her menstrual flows, which keeps her from school or participating in activities. If so, she could have endometriosis.

Endometriosis Present

This book is a concise magnum opus of current endometriosis information. It is a frank, comprehensive, and powerful key to unlocking the mysteries shrouding this perplexing disease. A conundrum for patients and healthcare providers alike, endometriosis is fraught with complexity and underappreciation.

Patients continue to face challenges in dealing with a society that does not recognize the word "endometriosis," much less fathom the experience of living with such an insidious illness. In an environment all too often characterized by misdiagnosis, substandard care, and drug-directed treatment focus, endometriosis continues to be handled with a tunnel vision approach, in which little has changed since the disease was first described by German physician Daniel Shroen more than 400 years ago. Many well-intentioned providers are simply unable to offer more to patients struggling with the illness, leaving them to suffer in silence. Fortunately, there is a better way, and it is entirely possible to triumph over endometriosis.

This is not just another book repeating the trite myths of the past. This book will let readers understand completely the basis for our current confusion and give hope for better treatment based on aggressively cutting out all disease instead of superficially burning it with lasers or treating symptoms with medicines. As more patients become educated about the disease, they will demand complete excision as the "gold standard" approach, and the number of gynecologic surgeons who advocate excision will increase.

A pioneer and world leader in the effective treatment of endometriosis for almost three decades, Dr. Redwine has set forth the highest standard for care, and patients are the ultimate beneficiaries. Upon reading this book, individuals with endometriosis will be armed with the information necessary to enable them to seek out optimal care through early intervention, accurate diagnosis, and effective treatment. Lighting up the darkness shrouding this illness, *100 Questions & Answers about Endometriosis* is crucial reading not only for patients, but for their loved ones and healthcare providers as well.

—Heather Guidone, Endometriosis Research Center

PART EIGHT

Final Thoughts

What treatments for endometriosis will
there be in the future?

Can endometriosis be prevented?

Will the confusion about endometriosis ever end?

More . . .

96. What treatments for endometriosis will there be in the future?

The failure of past medical therapies should not guide future therapies.

Who knows? Acquiring information about the genes involved in causing the disease may give us the first truly scientifically sound way of treating endometriosis without surgery—but this kind of treatment remains a long way off. The best hope for improved treatment of endometriosis in the foreseeable future is more widespread application of surgical excision of all disease. This is an achievable goal. Techniques exist for complete removal of endometriosis anywhere in the body. If a symptom is due to endometriosis, the symptom will disappear once the endometriosis is removed—it's that simple.

The problem is that there are very few surgeons in the world with all the skills necessary to treat endometriosis in every location. There are a few teams of multidisciplinary surgeons (including gynecologists, urologists, and bowel surgeons) who might be able to handle most cases of the disease. Beyond this, many general gynecologists have inadequate surgical skills for treating anything but the easiest cases.

The need for better surgical treatment of endometriosis could be helped by establishing centers of excellence in treating the disease. Such centers would attract both patients needing surgery and surgeons who want to learn to do the surgery. Another thing that would help would be to establish a subspecialty in the surgical treatment of endometriosis. Gynecology is already divided into several subspecialties—for example, maternal/fetal medicine, reproductive endocrinology, oncology, and urogynecology. Women with endometriosis outnumber the women who are helped by these established subspecialties, and everyone acknowledges how difficult endometriosis surgery can be. So why does gynecological cancer, a relatively uncommon disease treated by relatively simple surgery, have its own subspecialty? It can't be because of the skills required of the surgeons, so the difference must lie with the diagnosis itself: Cancer gets more respect than endometriosis. Endometriosis can't get no respect (to paraphrase Rodney Dangerfield).

97. Can endometriosis be prevented by medicine?

No.

98. Can endometriosis be prevented by surgery?

Possibly. If embryologically patterned metaplasia is the origin of endometriosis, then tracts of tissue that will form the disease are laid down during organogenesis, and the patterns and virulence of those tracts determined by many genes. The most common sites of these substrate tracts are across the cul-de-sac, uterosacral ligaments, and medial broad ligaments. These tracts extend to variable depths beneath the visible surface. If, at the first surgery done on a teenager, all of these areas are removed, even if they don't have endometriosis yet, then endometriosis might potentially be prevented because the susceptible substrate will have been removed before it developed into endometriosis. This is a hypothetical possibility that currently has no direct proof. However, it is clear from follow-up on patients who have undergone removal of endometriosis in these areas that the risk of surgery is small and the risk of postoperative adhesions is close to zero.

Surgical removal of the substrate tracts of tissue before they have formed endometriosis might potentially prevent the future development of endometriosis in those tracts.

99. What does the future hold for women with endometriosis?

Countless patients have suffered because of ineffective treatment that is directed against symptoms rather than the disease. The emphasis on medical therapy will continue because the fact that it is easier to prescribe medicine than to do the surgery necessary to treat endometriosis well.

Most obstetricians and gynecologists "participate" with insurance companies and many "participate" with **Medicare**, the federal health care program for older citizens. "Participation" means the doctors sign contracts with insurance companies or the federal government agreeing that the doctor will accept whatever amount of money the insurance company or Medicare deems necessary for doing surgery. Unfortunately, the system is designed in a way that these physicians don't get paid very much money to perform gynecological surgery.

The stark reality of this situation: if a surgeon is not paid to do surgery, surgery will frequently not be scheduled. Thus, if gynecologists perform less surgery, either their surgical skills will never fully develop or will remain in a perpetual state of rustiness. The end result is women with gynecological surgical needs, including those needing endometriosis surgery, may not get the high-quality surgery that they deserve.

As such, most specialists in endometriosis surgery decidedly do not accept *all* insurance plans, and some accept none. This gives them the economic and medical freedom to give their patients the best possible care. Considering the statistic that most women visit endometriosis surgeons only after having as many as

Medicare

A federal program in the United States that pays for health care for older citizens.

Doctors caring for pregnant women get more money than doctors caring for nonpregnant women.

15 previous surgeries, such patients may consider the higher fees charged by specialists in endometriosis surgery to be a small drop in the bucket.

100. Will the confusion about endometriosis ever end?

Yes, but only if Sampson's theory of reflux menstruation is completely abandoned and if better excisional surgery is available to more women.

Discarding Sampson's theory is necessary for the start of real progress in understanding endometriosis.

Endometriosis Future

The pain associated with endometriosis is not something women should be expected to live with—such pain is not normal! Yet, despite being described in the literature as far back as 1690, endometriosis did not get its present name until 1925, and old preconceptions about how the disease occurs and develops have yielded little progress in the last 80 years. Consequently, endometriosis remains an enigma where cure is difficult for the millions of women (and some men) across the globe who struggle with this disease on a daily basis.

The personal stories in this book illustrate perfectly the frustration that many women with endometriosis experience when they have to face multiple "hit-and-miss treatments." This continuation of ineffective treatments highlights the importance of individualized care and suggests that women must be referred to a center with the necessary expertise to offer all available treatments in a multidisciplinary context, including advanced laparoscopic surgery, which is already recognized by national boards of health in several European countries.

This book examines the benefits and flaws of current treatment regimens and provokes the reader to question the validity of some of the old assumptions. The author encourages the reader to think outside the box, which is not only healthy but essential when dealing with unsolved mysteries and enigmas.

100 Questions & Answers About Endometriosis offers fresh ideas and hypotheses that can help patients and physicians find new approaches to the treatment of endometriosis. Fresh viewpoints in terms of investigating disease origin, and subsequent treatment pathways, are particularly appropriate at a time where endometriosis has gained acceptance by the European Union as a disease that has a socioeconomic impact and a profound effect on a woman's quality of life. For women with endometriosis, the past has been a struggle, but the future looks brighter.

—Lone Hummelshoj, Publisher/Editor-in-Chief,
www.endometriosis.org

Additional Resources

A global forum for information about endometriosis:

www.endometriosis.org
The World Endometriosis Society: *www.endometriosis.ca*
The World Endometriosis Research Foundation:
www.endometriosisfoundation.org

Endometriosis Research Center (ERC)

This lay group provides education and up-to-date information about endometriosis. It is headquartered in Del Ray Beach, Florida.

www.endocenter.org
ERC.activeboard.com
www.endocenter.org/pdf/2008ScreeningEducationKit.pdf
groups.yahoo.com/group/mendomen
groups.yahoo.com/group/ERCGirlTalk

Endometriosis Association

This lay group is devoted to support, education, and research in the field of endometriosis. It is an international association with groups in many different countries. It is headquartered in Milwaukee, Wisconsin.

www.endometriosisassn.org

The EndoZONE

Endometriosis awareness and information

www.endometriosiszone.org

OBGYN.net

www.obgyn.net
wiki.obgyn.net/page/Endometriosis
forums.obgyn.net/endo

Endometriosis surgeons' websites

www.endometriosissurgeon.com
www.endometriosistreatment.org
www.centerforendo.com
www.reproductivecenter.com
www.pelvicpain.com
www.drcook.com
www.endoexcision.com
www.thomasllyons.com

Additional web resources

endoed.com
www.hcgresources.com/LapManual.pdf
www.hcgresources.com/endoindex.html
www.hcgresources.com/SurvivorLetter.html
www.endometriosis-uk.org/

Glossary

A

Ablation: Removal of diseased or unwanted tissue by surgery or other means.

Adeno-: A medical prefix that means relating to glandular tissue.

Adenomyoma: A benign nodular tumor composed of tissue containing glands and muscle. These tumors were first described in the uterus. Because deeply invasive endometriosis resembles an adenomyoma microscopically, "adenomyoma" was the first name given to what is now called deep endometriosis.

Adenomyosis: A benign disease of the uterus found more commonly in women after age 30. Glandular tissue from the lining of the uterus invades the muscle of the uterus. Symptoms include cramping uterine pain and bleeding.

Adhesion: A type of scar tissue that joins together two or more structures or surfaces which are normally separate.

Adhesiolysis: Surgically breaking or cutting adhesions.

Angiogenesis: Growth of new blood vessels (*angio-* means "blood").

Assisted reproductive technology (ART): Any technique that is used to enhance the chance of conception, such as in vitro fertilization (IVF) or intrauterine insemination (IUI).

Autotransplant: Tissue from one area of the body is transplanted surgically or by trauma to another part of the same body. In the new location, the tissue remains identical to tissue formerly in the previous location.

B

Bladder hydrodistention: A procedure for diagnosing interstitial cystitis in which an optical tube is inserted in the bladder, fluid is pumped into the bladder, the fluid is drained, and the physician then examines the bladder wall.

Bowel prep: A fluid that is more concentrated than normal intestinal contents and is used to prepare a person for bowel surgery. It creates an osmotic gradient that pulls water out of the bowel wall into the interior of the bowel, which flushes bowel contents along and out of the body. Bowel preps can be slightly dehydrating.

Bowel resection: The surgical removal of a portion of bowel. Bowel resections may be partial thickness, full thickness, or segmental.

C

Cecum: The beginning of the ascending colon, located on the lower right side of the abdomen. The appendix is attached to the cecum.

Cervix: The opening of the uterus through which menstrual blood passes. The cervix opens during labor and delivery to allow passage of the fetus out of the uterus during birth.

Corpus luteum cyst: A cyst formed by the ovary every month at the site of ovulation. Corpus luteum cysts can look just like endometrioma cysts on ultrasound or at surgery, but their pathological examination under a microscope can tell the difference.

Cul-de-sac: The bottom of the pelvis. It is the most common site of occurrence of endometriosis.

Cyst: A cavity filled with fluid. The fluid is not necessarily watery.

D

Deep endometriosis: Endometriosis that extends 5 mm or more beneath the visible pelvic surface.

Definitive diagnosis: A diagnosis that has been absolutely confirmed.

Differential diagnosis: A list of possible diagnoses based on the patient's history, physical exam and other tests; the doctor's best guess.

Dysmenorrhea: Painful menstrual flows. Not always in reference to uterine cramping.

Dyspareunia: Painful sexual intercourse.

E

Embryologically patterned metaplasia (EPM): A modern theory of origin of endometriosis. According to this theory, tracts of substrate tissue are laid down in the pelvis and elsewhere during formation of the embryo. After menarche (the first menstrual period), these tracts of tissue begin to change into endometriosis and the fibromuscular tissue that can surround some areas of endometriosis.

Endo-: A medical prefix meaning "inside" or "within."

Endometrioma: An ovarian cyst caused by endometriosis.

Endometriosis: A disease in which tissue that somewhat resembles the endometrium lining the uterine cavity is found outside the uterus where it doesn't belong. Symptoms include pain and sometimes infertility.

Endometrium: The tissue that lines the uterine cavity.

Estrogen: The main hormone produced by the ovaries.

Excision: To remove tissue surgically. Synonymous with resection.

F

Fallopian tubes: Hollow tubes that pick up eggs that have been released at ovulation and transport those eggs toward the uterus. Fertilization by a sperm occurs within the fallopian tube.

Fibroid: See *Uterine fibroid*.

Fimbriae: Hollow tubes that pick up eggs that have been released at ovulation and transport those eggs toward the uterus. Fertilization by a sperm occurs within the fallopian tube.

G

Gene: A segment of DNA carrying a code that directs a particular action to be taken by a cell.

Gene therapy: Replacing defective genes with normal genes to correct a disease state; or inserting a new gene that corrects the actions of a defective gene.

Glomerulation: A tiny area of capillary bleeding; a sign of interstitial cystitis.

GnRH agonists:
Gonadotropin-releasing hormone agonists; drugs that work by stimulating the pituitary gland so that it exhausts its ability to produce the hormones that stimulate the ovaries to produce estrogen. The initial stimulation of the ovaries may actually increase endometriosis pain in the first few weeks of treatment.

H

Heredity: The process by which genetic traits are passed from parents to their offspring.

Hormone: A molecule that is produced by one tissue and carried in the bloodstream to another tissue to cause a biological effect.

Hormone receptors: Sites on the surface of cells to which hormone molecules attach. The receptor sites are specific to a certain type of hormone. For example, estrogen receptors accept the attachment of estrogen; progesterone receptor accept the attachment of progesterone.

Hysterectomy: Surgical removal of the uterus.

I

Ileum: The second half of the small intestine.

Infertility: The state of being not fertile and unable to become pregnant.

Interstitial cystitis (IC): A condition of the urinary bladder in which the lining of the bladder has defects that allow the irritative contents of urine to bathe the bladder muscle directly.

Intracytoplasmic sperm injection (ICSI): A technique that forces fertilization of the egg by injecting sperm directly into the egg.

Intramural fibroid: A fibroid whose main volume arises from the middle of the muscular uterine wall.

Intrauterine (contraceptive) device (IUD): A small plastic device, sometimes impregnated with a progestin, that is placed inside the uterus to prevent pregnancy by interfering with implantation of the embryo.

Irritable bowel syndrome (IBS): A condition characterized by intestinal cramping, bloating, change in stool, nausea, diarrhea, and constipation. IBS may be caused by a disease such as endometriosis irritating the outside of the bowel, or it may have no identifiable cause.

L

Laparoscope: A small-diameter tube containing optical systems for transmitting illuminating light into the abdomen and the viewed image out of the abdomen.

Laparoscopy: The surgical use of a laparoscope to diagnose or treat disease.

Laparotomy: Opening the abdominal cavity with an incision made with a scalpel.

Laser: An acronym for "light amplification of stimulated emission radiation." In medical use refers to a high-powered, focused beam of light used to perform surgery.

M

Medicare: A federal program in the United States that pays for health care for older citizens.

Menstruation: The monthly discharge from the uterus; it consists of blood and endometrium sloughed from the uterine lining.

Metaplasia: A process by which one type of normal tissue changes into another type of tissue. Deeply invasive endometriosis is often surrounded by fibromuscular metaplasia.

Mucosa: A layer of tissue that has the ability to produce a secretion that can resemble mucus. The endometrium lining the interior of the uterus is a mucosal lining. Although the vagina doesn't have mucous glands in its wall, the transudate that it can produce is somewhat like mucous, so it is also a mucosa.

Myomectomy: Surgical removal of a fibroid from the uterus.

O

Obliteration of the cul-de-sac: A visual manifestation of severe endometriosis that can be seen at surgery. The rectum is stuck to the back of the cervix by scar tissue, so the normal cul-de-sac cannot be seen. This manifestation of endometriosis is associated with invasive disease of the uterosacral ligaments, cul-de-sac, and usually the front wall of the rectum. Invasion of the rear wall of the vagina sometimes occurs as well.

Ovarian hormones: The hormones produced by the ovaries: estrogen, progesterone, and testosterone.

Ovarian torsion: A condition in which an ovary twists around its blood supply.

Ovary: The repository for ova (eggs) inside the female.

Ovulation: The release of an ovum by an ovary. Sometimes more than one egg is released at ovulation.

Ovum: The medical term for an egg; plural = ova.

P

Pain management centers: Clinics in which several types of practitioners try to control the symptoms of endometriosis (and other pain-causing diseases) by using a multidisciplinary approach.

Pedunculated fibroid: A fibroid that hangs by a stalk from the outer surface of the uterus.

Peritoneal cavity: The internal bodily cavity lined by the peritoneum. This cavity contains the intestines, liver, spleen, and female pelvic organs.

Peritoneum: The shiny lining of the peritoneal cavity; resembles plastic kitchen wrap.

Posterior: An anatomical term. As a person is viewed standing, posterior is toward the back side of the body.

Progesterone: A hormone produced by the ovary, but only if ovulation has occurred. Its action is to prepare the endometrium for implantation of the embryo.

Progestin: An artificial hormone that has progesterone-like effects.

Pseudo-menopause: A hormonal state induced by GnRH agonists that somewhat mimics the hormonal state of menopause.

Pseudo-pregnancy: An artificial hormonal state resembling the hormonal state of pregnancy, induced by birth control pill therapy.

R

Randomized controlled trial (RCT): The "gold standard" of medical proof of the relative efficacy of one treatment over another, or over using nothing at all (placebo). Patients with a disease and who are similar to one another in most other respects (such as age, height, weight, duration of illness, and severity of disease) are assigned to one treatment group or another by randomization. The patients undergo treatment and are followed for a certain length of time to see if there is any difference in the results of the treatments studied.

Reflux menstruation: Menstrual blood exiting the uterus through the ends of the fallopian tubes rather than out through the cervix.

Renal agenesis: A urinary tract abnormality in which the kidney and ureter are missing on one side of the body.

Reproductive endocrinologist: A doctor who subspecializes in treatment to assist women in getting pregnant. After completing standard specialty training in obstetrics/gynecology, a physician completes an additional 2-year fellowship to become a reproductive endocrinologist.

Resection: To remove a piece of tissue surgically. Synonymous with excision.

S

Scar tissue: Fibrous tissue that forms as a result of healing of an injury or inflammation in the body.

Selection bias: A statistical term referring to skewed or unrepresentative results obtained due to the effect of using unusually specific or particular criteria to examine a group selected from a larger population.

Stent: (in ureteral surgery) a hollow plastic tube that ensures drainage of urine through the ureter into the bladder.

Submucosal fibroid: A fibroid that is next to the mucosa, the inner lining of the uterus.

Superficial endometriosis: Endometriosis that extends less than 5 mm beneath the visible pelvic surface.

T

Testosterone: A male hormone produced by the ovaries around the time of ovulation. It apparently increases the likelihood of mating and fertilization of eggs.

Trabeculation: A strand of bladder muscle that has become thicker than normal; a sign of interstitial cystitis.

U

Ureter: A hollow, muscular tube about the diameter of a pencil that drains urine from a kidney down into the bladder.

Uterine artery embolization (UAE): A procedure that shrinks the size of uterine fibroids by blocking the arteries to the fibroids, thereby depriving them of much of their blood supply.

Uterine fibroid (fibroid): A benign smooth muscle tumor arising from the muscular wall of the uterus.

Uterine lining: The interior lining of the uterus; the endometrium. The muscular wall of the uterus is the myometrium.

Uterus: The muscular organ that contains and supports the fetus before birth. The uterus has two parts: the upper body (fundus) and the opening (cervix).

Index